Introduction

Welcome to **"100+ Dishes of the Galveston Diet for Menopause,"** a culinary journey designed to empower and support women navigating the transformative stages of menopause. This book is a celebration of both delicious food and holistic health, offering a collection of nourishing recipes specifically crafted to align with the principles of the renowned Galveston Diet while addressing the unique nutritional needs of menopausal women.

Menopause marks a significant transition in a woman's life, characterized by hormonal fluctuations that can impact overall well-being, metabolism, and energy levels. As the body undergoes these changes, maintaining a balanced diet becomes paramount, not only for managing weight and energy but also for promoting hormonal harmony and supporting optimal health.

The Galveston Diet, founded by Dr. Mary Claire Haver, provides a holistic approach to nutrition, focusing on controlling insulin levels through a low-carbohydrate, high-healthy fat, and moderate-protein regimen. By emphasizing whole, nutrient-dense foods and minimizing processed ingredients, this dietary approach not only supports weight management and metabolic health but also fosters hormonal balance, which is crucial during menopause.

In this book, you'll find a diverse array of 105 recipes thoughtfully curated to offer delicious and satisfying meals that adhere to the principles of the Galveston Diet while catering to the nutritional needs of menopausal women. From vibrant salads to hearty mains and decadent desserts, each recipe is crafted to showcase the rich flavors of whole foods while providing essential nutrients to support hormonal health and overall well-being.

Whether you're seeking inspiration for nourishing breakfasts to start your day on the right foot, flavorful lunches to keep you energized, or comforting dinners to unwind after a busy day, you'll find a wealth of options within these pages. Each recipe is designed to be simple to prepare, allowing you to enjoy wholesome, homemade meals without sacrificing flavor or convenience.

As you embark on this culinary journey, I encourage you to embrace the transformative power of food and its ability to nurture your body, mind, and spirit during this significant stage of life. May these 105 dishes serve as a source of inspiration, nourishment, and vitality as you embrace the journey of menopause with grace, resilience, and delicious food.

Here's to vibrant health, hormonal harmony, and the joy of savoring every delicious bite along the way.

Bon appétit!

1. Grilled shrimp skewers with vegetables

Ingredients:
- 1 lb large shrimp, peeled and deveined
- 1 red bell pepper, cut into 1-inch pieces
- 1 yellow squash, sliced into 1/2-inch rounds
- 1 red onion, cut into 1-inch pieces
- 8-10 mushrooms, stems removed
- 1 pint cherry tomatoes
- 2 tbsp olive oil
- 2 tbsp lemon juice
- 2 cloves garlic, minced
- 1 tsp dried oregano
- Salt and pepper to taste
- Wooden or metal skewers, soaked if using wooden

Instructions:

1. In a large bowl, whisk together the olive oil, lemon juice, garlic, oregano and salt and pepper. Add the shrimp and vegetables and toss to coat evenly with the marinade. Cover and marinate for 30 minutes to 1 hour in the refrigerator.

2. Preheat grill to medium-high heat. Thread the shrimp and vegetables alternately onto the skewers, leaving a bit of space between pieces.

3. Grill the skewers for 2-3 minutes per side until the shrimp are opaque and the vegetables are tender but still crisp.

4. Transfer skewers to a platter and serve hot, with lemon wedges if desired.

You can mix up the vegetable varieties to your taste. The shrimp and veggie skewers make a great main course or appetizer!

2. Blackened fish tacos with cabbage slaw

Ingredients:
For the Fish:
- 1 lb firm white fish fillets (cod, mahi mahi, or tilapia)
- 2 tbsp blackening or Cajun seasoning
- 2 tbsp olive oil
- 8-10 small corn or flour tortillas, warmed

For the Slaw:
- 3 cups shredded cabbage
- 1/2 cup shredded carrots
- 1/4 cup chopped cilantro
- 3 tbsp lime juice
- 2 tbsp olive oil
- 1 tsp honey
- Salt and pepper to taste

Other Toppings:
- Diced avocado
- Lime wedges
- Sour cream or Mexican crema

Instructions:
1. Make the slaw by combining the shredded cabbage, carrots, cilantro, lime juice, olive oil, honey, and salt and pepper in a bowl. Toss to combine and set aside.

2. Pat the fish fillets dry and rub them all over with the blackening or Cajun seasoning.

3. Heat the olive oil in a skillet or grill pan over high heat. Add the seasoned fish and cook for 2-3 minutes per side until blackened and cooked through. Transfer to a plate and break into large flaky pieces.

4. Warm the tortillas according to package instructions.

5. To assemble the tacos, divide the fish among the tortillas and top with the cabbage slaw and desired toppings like avocado, sour cream and lime wedges.

For extra flavor, you can make a quick crema by combining 1/2 cup sour cream with 1-2 tbsp milk or cream, lime juice, salt and chopped cilantro.

These flavorful fish tacos with the crunchy slaw make a fun and tasty meal!

3. Baked salmon with dill sauce and roasted asparagus

Ingredients:
For the Salmon:
- 4 (6 oz) salmon fillets
- 2 tbsp olive oil
- Salt and pepper to taste

For the Dill Sauce:
- 1/2 cup sour cream
- 1/4 cup mayonnaise
- 2 tbsp fresh dill, chopped
- 2 tsp lemon juice
- 1 garlic clove, minced
- Salt and pepper to taste

For the Asparagus:
- 1 bunch asparagus, trimmed
- 2 tbsp olive oil
- Salt and pepper to taste

Instructions:
1. Preheat oven to 400°F. Line a baking sheet with foil or parchment paper.

2. Place the salmon fillets on the prepared baking sheet. Drizzle with olive oil and season with salt and pepper.

3. Bake for 12-15 minutes until salmon is opaque and flakes easily with a fork.

4. While the salmon bakes, make the dill sauce by combining the sour cream, mayonnaise, dill, lemon juice, garlic and salt/pepper in a small bowl.

5. On another baking sheet, toss the asparagus with olive oil and season with salt and pepper.

6. Roast the asparagus for 8-10 minutes until tender but still crisp.

7. Remove salmon and asparagus from oven. Serve the salmon warm, topped with the dill sauce alongside the roasted asparagus.

You can roast the asparagus at the same time as the salmon on a separate baking sheet for convenience. The fresh dill sauce adds such a bright vibrant flavor to the rich salmon.

4. Crab cakes with remoulade sauce

Ingredients:

For the Crab Cakes:
- 1 lb lump crabmeat, picked over for shells
- 1/4 cup panko breadcrumbs
- 2 green onions, thinly sliced
- 2 tbsp mayonnaise
- 1 egg, beaten
- 1 tbsp Dijon mustard
- 1 tbsp Worcestershire sauce
- 1 tsp Old Bay seasoning
- 2 tbsp butter for frying
- Lemon wedges for serving

For the Remoulade Sauce:
- 1/2 cup mayonnaise
- 2 tbsp Dijon mustard
- 2 tbsp ketchup
- 1 tbsp lemon juice
- 1 tbsp prepared horseradish
- 1 garlic clove, minced
- 1 tsp Worcestershire sauce
- 1 tsp paprika
- Hot sauce to taste
- Salt and pepper to taste

Instructions:

1. Make the remoulade first by whisking together all the sauce ingredients in a bowl until well-combined. Refrigerate until ready to use.

2. In a bowl, gently mix together the crabmeat, panko, green onions, mayonnaise, egg, mustard, Worcestershire and Old Bay until just combined, being careful not to overmix.

3. Form the crab mixture into 8 patties, using a 1/3 cup measuring cup to help get even portions.

4. In a skillet, heat the butter over medium heat. Cook the crab cakes for 3-4 minutes per side until golden brown and crispy on the outside.

5. Transfer crab cakes to a plate and serve warm with the remoulade sauce on the side and lemon wedges for squeezing over top.

For extra flavor, you can add some finely diced bell pepper, parsley or other herbs to the crab cake mixture. The cool, tangy remoulade sauce is the perfect pairing for the crispy crab cakes. Enjoy!

5. Seared ahi tuna over greens with citrus vinaigrette

Ingredients:

For the Tuna:
- 1 lb sashimi-grade ahi tuna steak
- 2 tsp olive oil
- Salt and pepper to taste

For the Salad:
- 5 oz mixed greens
- 1 avocado, sliced
- 1 grapefruit, segmented
- 1/4 red onion, thinly sliced

For the Citrus Vinaigrette:
- 1/4 cup olive oil
- 2 tbsp orange juice
- 1 tbsp lemon juice
- 1 tbsp lime juice
- 1 tsp honey
- 1 tsp Dijon mustard
- Salt and pepper to taste

Instructions:

1. Make the vinaigrette by whisking together the olive oil, orange juice, lemon juice, lime juice, honey, mustard, and salt/pepper in a small bowl or jar. Set aside.

2. Pat the tuna steak dry and season all over with salt and pepper.

3. Heat the olive oil in a skillet or grill pan over high heat until very hot. Sear the tuna for 1-2 minutes per side to get nicely browned on the outside while staying rare in the center.

4. Remove tuna from heat and let rest for 5 minutes before slicing against the grain into 1/4 inch thick slices.

5. Assemble the salads by dividing the mixed greens among plates. Top with avocado slices, grapefruit segments, and red onion slices.

6. Arrange the seared tuna slices over the top of each salad. Drizzle the citrus vinaigrette over the salads.

The contrast of the rare, meaty tuna with the fresh citrus vinaigrette, creamy avocado, and juicy grapefruit makes for such a flavorful and refreshing main course salad. Serve immediately after assembling for best results. Enjoy!

6. Shrimp and veggie stir fry over brown rice

Ingredients:
- 1 lb large shrimp, peeled and deveined
- 2 cups brown rice, cooked per package instructions
- 2 tbsp sesame oil
- 1 red bell pepper, sliced
- 1 cup broccoli florets
- 1 cup snow peas
- 1 cup sliced mushrooms
- 3 cloves garlic, minced
- 1 tbsp grated ginger
- 3 tbsp low-sodium soy sauce
- 2 tsp rice vinegar
- 1 tsp sesame seeds
- 2 green onions, sliced

Instructions:

1. Cook the brown rice per package instructions. Set aside when done.

2. In a large skillet or wok, heat the sesame oil over high heat. Add the bell pepper, broccoli, snow peas and mushrooms. Stir fry for 3-4 minutes.

3. Add the shrimp, garlic and ginger. Continue stir frying for 2 more minutes until shrimp starts to turn opaque.

4. Add the soy sauce and rice vinegar. Toss everything together and cook 1 more minute.

5. Remove from heat and stir in the sesame seeds and green onions.

6. Serve the shrimp and veggie stir fry immediately over the cooked brown rice.

For extra flavor, you can add a pinch of red pepper flakes or sriracha to the stir fry. Feel free to substitute in any veggies you like or have on hand like carrots, water chestnuts, bean sprouts etc. The fresh ginger adds such great aroma and flavor to this quick stir fry. Enjoy!

7. Baked stuffed flounder with spinach and feta

Ingredients:
- 4 (6-8 oz) flounder fillets
- 5 oz fresh spinach, chopped
- 1/2 cup crumbled feta cheese
- 1/4 cup panko breadcrumbs
- 2 tbsp fresh parsley, chopped
- 2 garlic cloves, minced
- 2 tbsp olive oil
- Zest of 1 lemon
- Salt and pepper to taste
- Lemon wedges for serving

Instructions:

1. Preheat oven to 400°F. Lightly grease a baking dish with cooking spray.

2. In a skillet, heat 1 tbsp olive oil over medium heat. Add the spinach and garlic and cook for 2-3 minutes until spinach is wilted. Remove from heat and let cool slightly.

3. In a bowl, mix together the cooked spinach, feta, panko, parsley, remaining 1 tbsp olive oil, lemon zest, and salt and pepper.

4. Pat the flounder fillets dry with a paper towel. Divide the spinach feta filling evenly among the fillets.

5. Roll or fold up the fillets to enclose the filling and secure with toothpicks if needed. Place the stuffed fillets seam-side down in the prepared baking dish.

6. Bake for 15-18 minutes until the fish is opaque and flakes easily with a fork.

7. Serve the baked stuffed flounder warm, garnished with lemon wedges to squeeze over top.

The bright lemon zest complements the rich, savory spinach and feta filling so nicely in this elegant baked fish dish. You can use any mild white fish like sole or tilapia for this recipe as well. Serve it with rice, potatoes or veggies on the side.

8. Grilled mahi mahi with pineapple salsa

Ingredients:

For the Mahi Mahi:
- 4 (6oz) mahi mahi fillets
- 2 tbsp olive oil
- 1 tsp chili powder
- 1 tsp cumin
- 1 tsp paprika
- Salt and pepper to taste

For the Pineapple Salsa:
- 1 cup diced pineapple
- 1/2 cup diced red bell pepper
- 1/4 cup diced red onion
- 2 tbsp chopped cilantro
- 2 tbsp lime juice
- 1 jalapeño, seeded and minced
- Salt to taste

Instructions:

1. Make the pineapple salsa by combining the pineapple, bell pepper, onion, cilantro, lime juice, jalapeño and salt in a bowl. Mix well and set aside.

2. Prepare the mahi mahi by brushing the fillets with olive oil and seasoning them evenly with the chili powder, cumin, paprika, salt and pepper.

3. Preheat grill or grill pan to medium-high heat and brush the grates with oil.

4. Grill the mahi mahi for 4-5 minutes per side until fish is opaque and flakes easily with a fork.

5. Transfer grilled mahi mahi to plates and top each fillet with a generous spoonful of the fresh pineapple salsa.

The sweet and tangy pineapple salsa pairs beautifully with the smoky spiced mahi mahi. You can make the salsa a few hours in advance to allow the flavors to meld.

Serve the grilled fish and salsa with some fresh lime wedges, rice or a salad on the side. The bright salsa adds such great fresh flavor to the grilled meaty mahi.

9. Seared scallops with wilted greens

Ingredients:
- 1 lb large sea scallops, patted very dry
- 2 tbsp olive oil, divided
- 2 tbsp butter, divided
- Salt and pepper
- 2 cloves garlic, minced
- 1 bunch Swiss chard or spinach, stems removed and chopped
- 1 bunch kale, stems removed and chopped
- 1 tbsp lemon juice
- Lemon wedges for serving

Instructions:

1. Pat the scallops very dry with paper towels and season both sides with salt and pepper.

2. Heat 1 tbsp each of olive oil and butter in a large skillet over high heat.

3. Once hot, add the scallops in a single layer and sear for 1-2 minutes per side until golden brown on both sides and opaque in the center. Remove scallops to a plate.

4. Reduce heat to medium, add remaining 1 tbsp each of olive oil and butter to the skillet.

5. Add the garlic and sauté for 30 seconds until fragrant.

6. Add the chopped greens and lemon juice. Toss and cook for 2-3 minutes, just until wilted.

7. Return the seared scallops and any accumulated juices to the skillet with the greens. Toss gently to combine.

8. Transfer the scallops and wilted greens to plates and serve immediately with lemon wedges for squeezing over top.

The sweet, caramelized seared scallops pair perfectly with the slightly bitter wilted greens. You can use a combination of greens like chard, kale, spinach or collards.

This makes an elegant yet healthy main course. Add a side of quinoa or rice if desired. The lemon juice brightens up the whole dish.

10. Shrimp and avocado salad

Ingredients:
- 1 lb cooked shrimp, peeled and deveined
- 2 avocados, diced
- 1 cup cherry tomatoes, halved
- 1/2 cup diced red onion
- 1/4 cup chopped cilantro
- 2 tbsp lime juice
- 2 tbsp olive oil
- 1 tbsp red wine vinegar
- 1 tsp honey
- 1 garlic clove, minced
- Salt and pepper to taste

Instructions:
1. In a large bowl, combine the cooked shrimp, diced avocados, cherry tomatoes, red onion, and cilantro.

2. In a small bowl, whisk together the lime juice, olive oil, red wine vinegar, honey, garlic, and salt and pepper to make the dressing.

3. Pour the dressing over the shrimp and avocado mixture and gently toss to coat everything evenly.

4. Let the salad sit for 10-15 minutes to allow flavors to meld.

5. Give it one more gentle toss, adjust seasoning if needed, and serve chilled or at room temperature.

Some optional add-ins include diced mango, corn, chopped jalapeño for heat, sliced hearts of palm, or crumbled queso fresco or feta cheese.

You can serve this salad as a main dish by portioning it over some greens, or as an appetizer with tortilla chips for scooping. The fresh flavors and creamy avocado pair so nicely with the shrimp.

11. Roasted brussels sprouts with bacon

Ingredients:
- 1 1/2 lbs brussels sprouts, trimmed and halved
- 4 slices thick-cut bacon, diced
- 2 tbsp olive oil
- 1 tbsp balsamic vinegar
- 2 cloves garlic, minced
- 1/4 tsp red pepper flakes (optional)
- Salt and pepper to taste

Instructions:

1. Preheat oven to 400°F. Line a baking sheet with foil or parchment paper.

2. Cut any large brussels sprouts in half and place them on the prepared baking sheet.

3. In a skillet over medium heat, cook the diced bacon until crispy. Transfer to a paper towel-lined plate, reserving about 2 tbsp of the bacon fat.

4. In a small bowl, whisk together the reserved 2 tbsp bacon fat, olive oil, balsamic vinegar, garlic, red pepper flakes if using, and salt and pepper.

5. Pour the bacon fat mixture over the brussels sprouts and toss to coat evenly.

6. Roast for 20-25 minutes, stirring halfway, until brussels sprouts are crispy and browned on the outside.

7. Remove from oven and transfer roasted brussels sprouts to a serving dish. Top with the crispy bacon pieces.

The brussels sprouts get delicious charred edges from the high oven temp. The bacon fat adds such great richness and the vinegar provides tangy contrast.

For extra flavor, you can add parmesan, pecans or dried cranberries before roasting. These roasted brussels sprouts make an exceptional side dish!

12. Grilled asparagus with lemon and parmesan

Ingredients:
- 1 1/2 lbs brussels sprouts, trimmed and halved
- 4 slices thick-cut bacon, diced
- 2 tbsp olive oil
- 1 tbsp balsamic vinegar
- 2 cloves garlic, minced
- 1/4 tsp red pepper flakes (optional)
- Salt and pepper to taste

Instructions:

1. Preheat oven to 400°F. Line a baking sheet with foil or parchment paper.

2. Cut any large brussels sprouts in half and place them on the prepared baking sheet.

3. In a skillet over medium heat, cook the diced bacon until crispy. Transfer to a paper towel-lined plate, reserving about 2 tbsp of the bacon fat.

4. In a small bowl, whisk together the reserved 2 tbsp bacon fat, olive oil, balsamic vinegar, garlic, red pepper flakes if using, and salt and pepper.

5. Pour the bacon fat mixture over the brussels sprouts and toss to coat evenly.

6. Roast for 20-25 minutes, stirring halfway, until brussels sprouts are crispy and browned on the outside.

7. Remove from oven and transfer roasted brussels sprouts to a serving dish. Top with the crispy bacon pieces.

The brussels sprouts get delicious charred edges from the high oven temp. The bacon fat adds such great richness and the vinegar provides tangy contrast.

For extra flavor, you can add parmesan, pecans or dried cranberries before roasting. These roasted brussels sprouts make an exceptional side dish! Let me know if you need any modifications.

13. Ratatouille (stewed summer vegetables)

Ingredients:
- 1 eggplant, diced into 1-inch cubes
- 1 zucchini, halved lengthwise and sliced into 1/2-inch pieces
- 1 yellow squash, halved lengthwise and sliced into 1/2-inch pieces
- 1 red bell pepper, diced into 1-inch pieces
- 1 yellow onion, diced
- 4 cloves garlic, minced
- 1 (14.5 oz) can diced tomatoes
- 2 tbsp olive oil
- 1 tsp dried thyme
- 1 tsp dried basil
- Salt and pepper to taste
- Fresh basil leaves, for garnish

Instructions:

1. Place the diced eggplant in a colander, sprinkle with salt and let sit for 30 minutes to draw out moisture. Rinse and pat dry.

2. In a large pot or dutch oven, heat the olive oil over medium heat. Add the onions and sauté for 5 minutes until translucent.

3. Add the garlic and cook for 1 minute until fragrant.

4. Add the zucchini, yellow squash, bell pepper, eggplant, diced tomatoes, thyme, basil, salt and pepper.

5. Bring the mixture to a simmer, then reduce heat to low. Let it stew for 30-45 minutes, stirring occasionally, until all the vegetables are very tender.

6. Adjust seasoning as needed, adding more salt, pepper, or fresh chopped basil. Serve warm.

Some optional additions are sliced olives, capers, or a pinch of red pepper flakes for heat. The ratatouille is delicious served over pasta, polenta, or with crusty bread.

It's a wonderfully rustic way to use peak summer veggies. The flavors deepen as the vegetables slowly stew together.

14. Cauliflower rice stir fry

Ingredients:
- 1 head cauliflower, riced (or 4 cups cauliflower rice)
- 2 tbsp sesame oil
- 1 cup broccoli florets
- 1 red bell pepper, sliced
- 1 cup snap peas or snow peas
- 3 cloves garlic, minced
- 1 tbsp grated ginger
- 2 eggs, beaten
- 3 tbsp low-sodium soy sauce
- 1 tsp rice vinegar
- 2 green onions, sliced
- Salt and pepper to taste

Instructions:

1. Prepare the cauliflower rice by grating a head of cauliflower with a box grater or pulsing florets in a food processor until rice-like in texture.

2. Heat 1 tbsp sesame oil in a large skillet or wok over medium-high heat. Add the riced cauliflower and stir-fry for 2-3 minutes until lightly crispy.

3. Push the cauliflower to the sides of the pan and add the beaten eggs in the center. Scramble the eggs, breaking them up into small pieces with a spatula, until cooked through.

4. Add in the remaining 1 tbsp sesame oil along with the broccoli, bell pepper, snap peas, garlic and ginger. Stir-fry for 3-4 minutes.

5. Add the soy sauce and rice vinegar. Toss everything to combine and cook 1 minute more.

6. Remove from heat and stir in the green onions. Season with salt and pepper to taste.

This is such a fresh, flavorful way to enjoy cauliflower rice. Feel free to use any variety of veggies you like or have on hand. The scrambled eggs add great protein.

You can also top it with cashews, sliced almonds or sesame seeds for some crunch. So quick and easy but full of nutrients!

15. Baked sweet potato fries

Ingredients:
- 3 large sweet potatoes, cut into 1/4-inch thick fries
- 2 tbsp olive oil
- 1 tsp salt
- 1/2 tsp black pepper
- 1/2 tsp garlic powder
- 1/2 tsp paprika
- 1/4 tsp cayenne pepper (optional for heat)

Instructions:

1. Preheat oven to 425°F. Line two large baking sheets with parchment paper or spray with non-stick cooking spray.

2. Rinse the cut sweet potato fries under cold water until the water runs clear to remove excess starch. This will help them get crispy. Pat them very dry with paper towels or a clean kitchen towel.

3. In a large bowl, toss the fries with the olive oil until evenly coated. Then sprinkle with the salt, black pepper, garlic powder, paprika, and cayenne if using. Toss again to coat evenly with the seasonings.

4. Spread the seasoned fries out in an even layer across the prepared baking sheets, leaving a bit of space between them.

5. Bake for 15 minutes, then flip the fries over with a spatula. Bake for 10-15 minutes more until crispy and browned.

6. Remove from oven and let cool 5 minutes before serving. The fries will crisp up more as they cool. Serve warm with your favorite dipping sauces like ketchup, ranch, BBQ, etc.

The trick is to cut the fries into thin, even strips and bake at a high temp after tossing with just a little oil. This concentrates their natural sweet flavor. So addictive and healthier than fried! Enjoy.

16. Zucchini noodles with marinara

Ingredients:
- 4 medium zucchinis
- 1 tbsp olive oil
- 3 garlic cloves, minced
- 1 (24 oz) jar marinara sauce
- 1/4 cup fresh basil leaves, chopped
- 2 tbsp grated parmesan, plus more for serving
- Salt and pepper to taste

Instructions:

1. Use a spiralizer, julienne peeler, or sharp knife to cut the zucchinis into long, thin noodle-like strips. Place zucchini noodles in a colander and sprinkle with salt. Let sit for 15-30 minutes to drain excess moisture.

2. Heat the olive oil in a large skillet over medium heat. Add the garlic and cook for 1 minute until fragrant.

3. Add the marinara sauce and season with salt and pepper to taste. Simmer for 5 minutes.

4. Pat the zucchini noodles dry with paper towels or a clean kitchen towel. Add them to the sauce and toss gently for 2-3 minutes until slightly softened but still retaining a crisp texture.

5. Remove from heat and stir in the fresh basil and parmesan cheese.

6. Serve the zucchini noodles immediately, topped with extra parmesan cheese if desired.

The zucchini noodles make a light, low-carb alternative to pasta. But they still allow you to enjoy the flavors of a classic marinara sauce.

For extra protein, you can add cooked chicken, shrimp or ground turkey/beef to the sauce. You can also toss in sauteed veggies like spinach, bell peppers or mushrooms.

17. Sauteed spinach with garlic

Ingredients:
- 2 tablespoons olive oil
- 3 cloves garlic, minced
- 2 bunches fresh spinach, washed and stems trimmed
- 1/4 teaspoon red pepper flakes (optional)
- 1 tablespoon lemon juice
- Salt and pepper to taste

Instructions:

1. In a large skillet or sauté pan, heat the olive oil over medium heat. Add the minced garlic and red pepper flakes (if using). Sauté for 1 minute until garlic is fragrant but not browned.

2. Add the spinach to the pan in batches if needed, letting it wilt down before adding more. Use tongs to gently toss and coat the spinach with the garlic-olive oil mixture.

3. Continue sautéing for 2-3 minutes, tossing frequently, until spinach is completely wilted.

4. Remove from heat and squeeze the lemon juice over top. Give it one final toss to combine.

5. Season with salt and pepper to taste.

6. Transfer sauteed spinach to a serving bowl or plate. Optionally garnish with extra red pepper flakes or lemon wedges.

You want to avoid overcooking the spinach so it retains its bright green color and doesn't get too soggy.

This makes a flavorful, healthy side dish. Or you can serve it as a bed for proteins like fish, chicken or steak. The garlic aroma is irresistible!

18. Roasted beet and arugula salad

Ingredients:
- 4-5 medium beets, greens removed
- 2 tablespoons olive oil
- Salt and pepper
- 5 oz arugula
- 1/2 cup crumbled goat or feta cheese
- 1/4 cup toasted walnuts or pecans
- 2 tablespoons balsamic vinegar
- 1 tablespoon dijon mustard
- 2 tablespoons olive oil
- 1 clove garlic, minced

Instructions:

1. Preheat oven to 400°F. Scrub beets and trim stems down to 1 inch. Toss beets with 2 tbsp olive oil and sprinkle with salt and pepper. Wrap in foil and roast for 45-60 minutes until tender when pierced with a fork.

2. Allow roasted beets to cool slightly, then peel off skins and cut into wedges or chunks.

3. Make the dressing by whisking together the balsamic vinegar, mustard, 2 tbsp olive oil, garlic and a pinch each of salt and pepper.

4. Place the arugula in a large bowl and toss with just enough dressing to lightly coat the leaves.

5. Add the roasted beet pieces, crumbled cheese and toasted nuts to the arugula.

6. Drizzle any remaining dressing over the top and toss gently to combine.

7. Serve the salad immediately while the beets are still warm for best flavor.

You can adjust amounts of dressing, cheese and nuts to taste preference. This makes a flavorful salad with the earthiness of the beets complemented by the peppery arugula, tangy dressing and creamy cheese.

19. Stuffed bell peppers with quinoa

Ingredients:
- 6 bell peppers (any color), tops cut off and seeds/membranes removed
- 1 cup uncooked quinoa, rinsed
- 2 cups vegetable or chicken broth
- 1 tablespoon olive oil
- 1 onion, diced
- 2 cloves garlic, minced
- 1 cup cooked black beans or pinto beans, drained and rinsed
- 1 cup corn kernels (fresh or frozen)
- 1/2 cup shredded cheese (cheddar, monterey jack, etc)
- 2 tablespoons chopped fresh cilantro or parsley
- 1 teaspoon cumin
- 1 teaspoon chili powder
- Salt and pepper to taste
- Salsa or enchilada sauce for serving (optional)

Instructions:
1. Preheat oven to 375°F. Arrange hollowed out bell pepper halves in a baking dish and set aside.

2. In a saucepan, combine quinoa and broth. Bring to a boil, then reduce heat and simmer covered for 15-20 minutes until liquid is absorbed. Fluff with a fork.

3. In a skillet, heat the olive oil over medium heat. Sauté the onion for 2-3 minutes until translucent. Add the garlic and cook 1 minute more.

4. Transfer cooked quinoa to a bowl and stir in the sautéed onion/garlic, black beans, corn, cheese, cilantro, cumin, chili powder and salt/pepper to taste. Mix well.

5. Stuff the quinoa mixture into the bell pepper halves, packing it in firmly and mounding it on top.

6. Pour a small amount of broth or water into the bottom of the baking dish. Cover with foil.

7. Bake for 30 minutes, then uncover and bake 15 minutes more until peppers are tender. Serve the stuffed peppers warm, drizzled with salsa or enchilada sauce if desired.

You can easily make this vegan by omitting the cheese or using a vegan cheese substitute. You can also mix up the fillings with different veggies, beans or spices. Quinoa makes a delicious protein-packed stuffing!

20. Grilled vegetable kabobs

Ingredients:
- 1 zucchini, cut into 1-inch pieces
- 1 yellow squash, cut into 1-inch pieces
- 1 red bell pepper, cut into 1-inch pieces
- 1 red onion, cut into 1-inch pieces
- 8 oz mushrooms, left whole if small or cut in half
- 1 pint cherry or grape tomatoes
- Wooden or metal skewers
- 2 tablespoons olive oil
- 2 tablespoons balsamic vinegar
- 2 cloves garlic, minced
- 1 teaspoon dried oregano
- 1/2 teaspoon salt
- 1/4 teaspoon black pepper

Marinade:
- 1/4 cup olive oil
- 2 tablespoons balsamic vinegar
- 2 cloves garlic, minced
- 1 teaspoon dried basil
- 1 teaspoon dried oregano
- 1/2 teaspoon salt
- 1/4 teaspoon black pepper

Instructions:

1. If using wooden skewers, soak them in water for 30 minutes to prevent burning.

2. In a large bowl, whisk together the marinade ingredients. Add the prepped vegetables and toss to coat evenly in the marinade. Cover and marinate for 30 minutes.

3. Preheat grill to medium-high heat. Thread the marinated vegetables onto the skewers in an alternating pattern.

4. In a small bowl, whisk together the olive oil, balsamic vinegar, garlic, oregano, salt and pepper.

5. Brush or spray the vegetable kabobs with the olive oil mixture on all sides.

6. Grill the kabobs for 12-15 minutes, turning every few minutes, until vegetables are tender and slightly charred.

7. Brush or drizzle with any remaining olive oil mixture from the bowl.

8. Serve the vegetable kabobs warm, garnished with chopped parsley if desired.

You can mix and match your favorite veggies on the skewers. Some other great options are eggplant, potatoes, beets or brussels sprouts. The marinade helps add flavor while the olive oil mix prevents sticking and charring on the grill.

21. Lemon rosemary chicken

Ingredients:
- 4 boneless, skinless chicken breasts
- 1⁄4 cup olive oil
- 1⁄3 cup freshly squeezed lemon juice (about 2 lemons)
- Zest of 1 lemon
- 3 cloves garlic, minced
- 2 tablespoons fresh rosemary, finely chopped
- 1 teaspoon salt
- 1⁄2 teaspoon black pepper
- 1 lemon, thinly sliced into rounds

Instructions:
1. In a shallow dish, whisk together the olive oil, lemon juice, lemon zest, garlic, rosemary, salt and pepper.

2. Add the chicken breasts and turn to coat both sides in the marinade. Cover and marinate for at least 30 minutes at room temperature, or up to overnight in the refrigerator.

3. Preheat oven to 400°F.

4. Remove chicken from marinade and place in a baking dish. Pour any remaining marinade over the top.

5. Arrange the lemon slices on top and around the chicken pieces.

6. Bake for 25-35 minutes, basting once or twice with the pan juices, until chicken is cooked through (165°F internal temp).

7. Allow chicken to rest 5 minutes before serving.

8. Transfer chicken to plates and spoon the pan juices with garlic, rosemary and lemon over the top.

For extra flavor, you can sear the chicken first in a hot skillet with some of the marinade before baking. The lemon slices add a bright, fresh taste and keep the chicken incredibly tender and juicy.

You can easily double or triple the ingredients for more servings. Serve this with roasted potatoes or rice and a salad or vegetable side for a complete meal.

22. Turkey lettuce wraps

Ingredients:
- 4 boneless, skinless chicken breasts
- 1⁄4 cup olive oil
- 1⁄3 cup freshly squeezed lemon juice (about 2 lemons)
- Zest of 1 lemon
- 3 cloves garlic, minced
- 2 tablespoons fresh rosemary, finely chopped
- 1 teaspoon salt
- 1⁄2 teaspoon black pepper
- 1 lemon, thinly sliced into rounds

Instructions:

1. In a shallow dish, whisk together the olive oil, lemon juice, lemon zest, garlic, rosemary, salt and pepper.

2. Add the chicken breasts and turn to coat both sides in the marinade. Cover and marinate for at least 30 minutes at room temperature, or up to overnight in the refrigerator.

3. Preheat oven to 400°F.

4. Remove chicken from marinade and place in a baking dish. Pour any remaining marinade over the top.

5. Arrange the lemon slices on top and around the chicken pieces.

6. Bake for 25-35 minutes, basting once or twice with the pan juices, until chicken is cooked through (165°F internal temp).

7. Allow chicken to rest 5 minutes before serving.

8. Transfer chicken to plates and spoon the pan juices with garlic, rosemary and lemon over the top.

For extra flavor, you can sear the chicken first in a hot skillet with some of the marinade before baking. The lemon slices add a bright, fresh taste and keep the chicken incredibly tender and juicy.

You can easily double or triple the ingredients for more servings. Serve this with roasted potatoes or rice and a salad or vegetable side for a complete meal.

23. Grilled pork tenderloin with apples

Ingredients:
- 1 pork tenderloin (around 1 to 1.25 lbs)
- 2 tablespoons olive oil
- 2 cloves garlic, minced
- 1 tablespoon fresh rosemary, chopped
- 1 teaspoon salt
- 1/2 teaspoon black pepper
- 2 apples (gala, fuji or honeycrisp), cut into 1/2 inch wedges
- 2 tablespoons butter
- 2 tablespoons brown sugar
- 1/2 teaspoon ground cinnamon

Instructions:
1. In a small bowl, combine the olive oil, minced garlic, rosemary, salt and pepper. Rub the mixture all over the pork tenderloin. Cover and marinate for 30 minutes at room temperature.

2. Preheat grill to medium-high heat (375°F-400°F).

3. Make an aluminum foil packet for the apple wedges: Place apples in the center of a sheet of foil. Top with butter, brown sugar and cinnamon. Seal the packet closed.

4. Grill the pork tenderloin for 15-20 minutes, turning occasionally, until internal temperature reaches 145°F on a meat thermometer.

5. During the last 10 minutes of grilling, place the foil apple packet on the grill grates and heat until the apples are softened.

6. Transfer the grilled pork to a cutting board and let rest for 5 minutes before slicing.

7. Open the apple packet and transfer the apple wedges and sauce to a bowl.

8. Slice the pork tenderloin into 1/2-inch pieces and serve hot, topped with the grilled cinnamon apples.

The sweetness of the brown sugar glazed apples perfectly complements the savory herb pork tenderloin. You can also grill some thick onion slices alongside for extra flavor.

Serve this with roasted potatoes or garlic mashed potatoes and a side salad or vegetable for a complete and impressive meal.

24. Beef and vegetable stir fry

Ingredients:
- 1 lb flank steak or sirloin,
  thinly sliced across the grain
- 2 tablespoons vegetable oil, divided
- 2 cups broccoli florets
- 1 red bell pepper, sliced
- 1 cup sliced mushrooms
- 1 small onion, sliced
- 2 cloves garlic, minced
- 1 teaspoon grated fresh ginger
- 1/4 cup low-sodium soy sauce
- 2 tablespoons rice vinegar
- 1 tablespoon brown sugar
- 1 teaspoon sesame oil
- 1/4 teaspoon red pepper flakes (optional)
- 3 cups cooked rice, for serving

Instructions:

1. In a small bowl, whisk together the soy sauce, rice vinegar, brown sugar, sesame oil and red pepper flakes (if using). Set aside.

2. Heat 1 tablespoon of vegetable oil in a large skillet or wok over high heat. Add the sliced beef and stir-fry for 2-3 minutes until browned but not fully cooked through. Transfer beef to a plate.

3. Add the remaining 1 tablespoon of oil to the skillet. Add the broccoli, bell pepper, mushrooms and onion. Stir-fry for 4-5 minutes until vegetables are crisp-tender.

4. Add the minced garlic and grated ginger. Stir-fry for 30 seconds until fragrant.

5. Return the beef and any accumulated juices back to the skillet with the vegetables.

6. Whisk the sauce again to recombine and pour over the beef and vegetables. Toss to coat everything evenly.

7. Allow to simmer for 1-2 minutes to heat through and thicken the sauce slightly. Serve the beef and vegetable stir-fry immediately over steamed rice.

Some optional additions are sliced water chestnuts, snap peas, baby corn or bean sprouts for extra crunch and vegetables. You can also substitute the protein with chicken, shrimp or tofu if desired.

The keys are thinly sliced meat, cooking over very high heat in batches so ingredients don't overcrowd the pan, and tossing frequently. This allows you to get the signature smoky "wok-charred" flavor in the stir-fry.

25. Bison burgers with avocado

Ingredients:
- 1 lb ground bison meat
- 1 egg, lightly beaten
- 1/4 cup breadcrumbs
- 2 cloves garlic, minced
- 1 tsp smoked paprika
- 1 tsp ground cumin
- 1 tsp dried oregano
- 1/2 tsp salt
- 1/4 tsp black pepper
- 4 burger buns, lightly toasted
- 1 avocado, pitted and sliced
- Desired toppings like lettuce, tomato, onion etc.

Instructions:

1. In a bowl, mix together the ground bison, egg, breadcrumbs, garlic, paprika, cumin, oregano, salt and pepper until well combined. Be careful not to overmix.

2. Divide the mixture into 4 equal patties, about 1/2 inch thick. Make a slight indentation in the center of each patty to prevent excessive doming during cooking.

3. Preheat grill or grill pan to medium-high heat and brush with oil.

4. Grill the bison burgers for 4-5 minutes per side for medium doneness, adjusting time for desired level of cooking.

5. During the last 1-2 minutes of cooking, lightly toast the buns on the grill.

6. Remove burgers from grill and allow to rest for 5 minutes.

7. Assemble the burgers by placing on bun bottoms then topping each with sliced avocado and any other desired toppings like lettuce, tomato, onion, etc.

8. Spread bun tops with mayonnaise, mustard or other desired condiments and place on top.

Bison is a lean meat with a delicious rich flavor. The avocado adds a buttery, creamy contrast. You can customize with your favorite burger toppings.

For extra flavor, mix together mayo, garlic, lemon juice and fresh herbs to slather on the buns and burger patties. Serve with a side of sweet potato fries, salad or grilled veggies for a tasty meal!

26. Mediterranean chicken kebabs

Ingredients:
- 1 lb boneless, skinless chicken breasts, cut into 1-inch chunks
- 1 red bell pepper, cut into 1-inch pieces
- 1 red onion, cut into 1-inch chunks
- 8oz whole mushrooms
- 1 zucchini, cut into 1/2-inch thick rounds
- Wooden or metal skewers

Yogurt Sauce (optional):
- 1 cup plain Greek yogurt
- 1 clove garlic, minced
- 1 tablespoon lemon juice
- 1/4 cup chopped fresh parsley or dill
- Salt and pepper to taste

Marinade:
- 1/4 cup olive oil
- 3 tablespoons lemon juice
- 3 garlic cloves, minced
- 2 teaspoons dried oregano
- 1 teaspoon dried basil
- 1 teaspoon paprika
- 1/2 teaspoon salt
- 1/4 teaspoon black pepper

Instructions:

1. If using wooden skewers, soak them in water for 30 minutes before threading.

2. In a shallow dish, whisk together all the marinade ingredients. Add the chicken and vegetables and toss to coat well. Cover and marinate for 30 mins to 1 hour.

3. Thread the marinated chicken, vegetables and mushrooms alternately onto the skewers in a pattern. Discard remaining marinade.

4. Preheat grill to medium-high heat. Grill the kebabs for 12-15 minutes, turning every few minutes, until chicken is cooked through and vegetables are tender.

5. For the yogurt sauce (if using), mix together the yogurt, garlic, lemon juice, parsley/dill and salt/pepper.

6. Serve the Mediterranean chicken kebabs with yogurt sauce on the side for dipping or drizzling over top.

The aromatic lemon-herb marinade infuses the chicken and veggies with so much fresh Mediterranean flavor. The cool yogurt sauce complements it perfectly.

You can easily customize by swapping in your preferred veggies like tomatoes, eggplant, artichokes or even fruits like pineapple. Brushing the kebabs with marinade while grilling adds even more caramelized flavor.

27. Garlic shrimp fajitas

Ingredients:
- 1 lb large shrimp, peeled and deveined
- 2 tablespoons olive oil
- 4 cloves garlic, minced
- 1 teaspoon chili powder
- 1 teaspoon ground cumin
- 1/2 teaspoon smoked paprika
- 1/4 teaspoon cayenne pepper (optional for heat)
- 1 red bell pepper, sliced
- 1 green bell pepper, sliced
- 1 large onion, sliced
- Juice of 1 lime
- Salt and pepper to taste
- 8-10 small flour or corn tortillas
- Toppings like shredded cheese, salsa, guacamole, sour cream, etc.

Instructions:

1. Pat the shrimp dry and season with salt, pepper, and a pinch of the chili powder and cumin.

2. Heat the olive oil in a large skillet or griddle pan over high heat. Add the shrimp and garlic and sauté for 2-3 minutes until shrimp starts to turn opaque. Remove shrimp to a plate.

3. In the same pan, add the sliced bell peppers and onions. Sauté for 5-6 minutes until starting to char and soften slightly.

4. Add the remaining chili powder, cumin, paprika, cayenne (if using), and lime juice. Toss to coat the veggies in the spices.

5. Return the shrimp and any accumulated juices to the pan. Toss everything together and cook for 1-2 more minutes until shrimp is fully cooked through.

6. Warm the tortillas by wrapping in foil and placing in the oven at 350°F for 5-10 minutes until heated through.

7. Serve the shrimp and veggie fajita mixture with the warm tortillas, shredded cheese, salsa, guacamole, sour cream and any other desired toppings.

The garlic shrimp get a punch of flavor from the zesty spice blend. The lime juice adds fantastic brightness to the charred veggies.

You can easily make this recipe for just 2 people or scale it up for larger crowds. It's a healthier take on fajitas that is fast, fresh and delicious! Serve with Mexican rice and beans on the side.

28. Tofu veggie stir fry

Ingredients:
- 14 oz extra-firm tofu, drained and cubed
- 2 tablespoons soy sauce or tamari, divided
- 2 tablespoons rice vinegar, divided
- 2 tablespoons sesame oil, divided
- 1 tablespoon cornstarch
- 1 red bell pepper, sliced
- 1 cup broccoli florets
- 1 cup sliced mushrooms
- 1 cup snap or snow peas
- 3 cloves garlic, minced
- 1 tablespoon freshly grated ginger
- 3 green onions, sliced, whites and greens separated
- Cooked rice or noodles, for serving

***Sauce*:**
- 1/4 cup vegetable or chicken broth
- 2 tablespoons soy sauce or tamari
- 1 tablespoon rice vinegar
- 1 teaspoon sesame oil
- 2 teaspoons brown sugar
- 1 teaspoon cornstarch
- 1/4 teaspoon red pepper flakes (optional)

Instructions:

1. In a small bowl, toss the cubed tofu with 1 tablespoon each soy sauce, rice vinegar and sesame oil. Sprinkle with 1 tablespoon cornstarch and toss to coat evenly.

2. Make the sauce by whisking together all the sauce ingredients in a separate bowl until combined. Set aside.

3. Heat 1 tablespoon sesame oil in a large skillet or wok over high heat. Add the marinated tofu and fry for 2-3 minutes until lightly browned on the outside. Transfer to a plate.

4. Add the remaining 1 tablespoon sesame oil to the skillet/wok. Add the bell pepper, broccoli, mushrooms, snap peas and whites of the green onions. Stir fry for 3-4 minutes.

5. Add the garlic, ginger and remaining 1 tablespoon each soy sauce and rice vinegar. Stir fry for 1 minute more.

6. Whisk the sauce again to recombine, then pour it into the veggie mixture. Add the fried tofu back in as well.

7. Cook while tossing frequently for 2-3 minutes until sauce thickens slightly and vegetables are crisp-tender.

8. Remove from heat and stir in the green onion greens. Serve immediately over steamed rice or noodles.

The tofu gets a nice crispy coating from the cornstarch before being added to the flavorful stir fried veggies in a savory garlic-ginger sauce.

Feel free to substitute or add in any other veggie favorites like carrots, cabbage, eggplant or baby corn. You can also swap the tofu for chicken, shrimp or beef if preferred. This makes a nutritious and delicious plant-based meal!

29. Turkey meatballs in marinara

Ingredients:
Meatballs:
- 1 lb ground turkey
- 1 egg
- 1/2 cup breadcrumbs
- 1/4 cup grated parmesan cheese
- 2 cloves garlic, minced
- 2 tablespoons fresh parsley, chopped
- 1 teaspoon Italian seasoning
- 1/2 teaspoon salt
- 1/4 teaspoon black pepper

Marinara Sauce:
- 1 tablespoon olive oil
- 1 onion, diced
- 3 garlic cloves, minced
- 1 (28oz) can crushed tomatoes
- 1 (6oz) can tomato paste
- 2 teaspoons Italian seasoning
- 1 teaspoon sugar
- 1/4 cup fresh basil, chopped
- Salt and pepper to taste

Instructions:
1. For the meatballs: In a bowl, mix together the turkey, egg, breadcrumbs, parmesan, garlic, parsley, Italian seasoning, salt and pepper until well combined. Roll into 1-inch balls.

2. In a large skillet, heat olive oil over medium-high heat. Add the meatballs in batches and cook for 2-3 minutes per batch until browned on all sides. Transfer to a plate.

3. For the marinara: In the same skillet, add the onion and cook for 3-4 minutes until translucent. Add the garlic and cook for 1 minute until fragrant.

4. Add the crushed tomatoes, tomato paste, Italian seasoning, sugar and basil. Season with salt and pepper to taste.

5. Return the browned meatballs to the skillet and submerge into the marinara sauce. Reduce heat to low, cover and simmer for 20-25 minutes, stirring occasionally, until meatballs are fully cooked through.

6. Serve the turkey meatballs in marinara sauce over cooked pasta, zucchini noodles, mashed cauliflower or crusty bread for dipping. Garnish with extra parmesan and basil.

The lean turkey meatballs are bursting with flavor from the herbs and parmesan. Simmering them in the rich and rustic marinara sauce makes them incredibly tender and tasty.

You can easily double this recipe to have extra meatballs for meal prepping or freezing extras for later. A side salad and garlic bread complete this comforting Italian dinner!

30. Grilled chicken souvlaki salad

Ingredients:
- 1 lb boneless, skinless chicken breasts,
cut into 1-inch cubes
- 2 tablespoons olive oil
- 2 tablespoons lemon juice
- 2 cloves garlic, minced
- 1 teaspoon dried oregano
- 1/2 teaspoon salt
- 1/4 teaspoon black pepper
- 6 cups chopped romaine lettuce
- 1 cup cherry tomatoes, halved
- 1 cucumber, diced
- 1/2 red onion, thinly sliced
- 1/2 cup crumbled feta cheese
- 1/4 cup pitted kalamata olives

Dressing:
- 1/4 cup olive oil
- 2 tablespoons red wine vinegar
- 1 tablespoon lemon juice
- 1 clove garlic, minced
- 1 teaspoon dried oregano
- 1/2 teaspoon Dijon mustard
- Salt and pepper to taste

Instructions:

1. In a shallow dish, combine the 2 tbsp olive oil, 2 tbsp lemon juice, 2 cloves minced garlic, 1 tsp oregano, salt and pepper. Add the cubed chicken and toss to coat. Cover and marinate for 30 minutes to 1 hour.

2. Soak wooden skewers in water for 30 mins if using. Thread the marinated chicken onto the skewers.

3. Preheat grill or grill pan to medium-high heat. Grill the chicken skewers for 8-10 minutes, turning occasionally, until chicken is cooked through.

4. Make the dressing by whisking together the 1/4 cup olive oil, 2 tbsp red wine vinegar, 1 tbsp lemon juice, 1 clove garlic, 1 tsp oregano, 1/2 tsp Dijon, and salt & pepper to taste.

5. In a large bowl, combine the chopped romaine, cherry tomatoes, cucumber, red onion, feta and olives. Remove chicken from skewers and cut any larger pieces in half.

6. Add the grilled chicken to the salad bowl and drizzle with the desired amount of dressing. Toss to combine. Serve the souvlaki salad garnished with extra feta and a lemon wedge if desired.

The bright, tangy flavors in the dressing pair perfectly with the charred chicken, crisp veggies, salty feta and briny olives. This makes a protein-packed, Mediterranean-inspired meal salad.

For extra crunch you can add garbanzo beans, radishes or croutons. You can also serve the salad components separately with pita bread on the side. It's healthy, satisfying and full of fresh summertime flavors!

31. Seafood gumbo

Ingredients:
- 1/2 cup vegetable oil
- 1/2 cup all-purpose flour
- 1 large onion, diced
- 1 green bell pepper, diced
- 2 celery ribs, diced
- 4 cloves garlic, minced
- 1 tablespoon Cajun or Creole seasoning
- 2 bay leaves
- 4 cups seafood or fish stock
- 1 (14.5 oz) can diced tomatoes
- 1 pound shrimp, peeled and deveined
- 1 pound lump crabmeat or crawfish tails
- 8 oz andouille or smoked sausage, sliced
- 2 tablespoons Worcestershire sauce
- 2 tablespoons fresh parsley, chopped
- 4 green onions, sliced
- Steamed rice, for serving

Instructions:

1. In a large heavy-bottomed pot or dutch oven, make the roux by heating the oil over medium heat. Whisk in the flour and cook, stirring constantly, until the roux is brick red in color, about 15-20 minutes. Be careful not to burn it.

2. Add the onions, bell pepper and celery. Cook for 5 minutes until vegetables are softened.

3. Add the garlic and Cajun seasoning and cook for 1 minute until fragrant.

4. Gradually whisk in the stock and tomatoes. Add the bay leaves. Bring to a boil, then reduce heat and simmer for 30 minutes, stirring occasionally.

5. Add the shrimp, crabmeat, sausage and Worcestershire sauce. Simmer for 10 minutes until shrimp is cooked through.

6. Remove bay leaves. Stir in the parsley and green onions.

7. Taste and adjust seasoning as needed with salt, pepper, Cajun seasoning or more Worcestershire.

8. Serve the seafood gumbo over steamed rice, garnished with extra green onions if desired.

The key is cooking the roux slowly until it gets a deep, rich color and nutty flavor. This gives the gumbo its signature thick, velvety texture. For extra richness, you can let the shrimp shells simmer in the stock for 30 minutes before straining and using the stock.

Oysters, crab claws or fish like cod can also be added. Let the gumbo sit for a few hours to allow the flavors to meld for the best taste. Serve with crusty French bread or cornbread on the side.

32. Chicken vegetable soup

Ingredients:
- 1 tablespoon olive oil
- 1 onion, diced
- 3 carrots, peeled and sliced
- 3 celery ribs, sliced
- 3 cloves garlic, minced
- 8 cups chicken broth
- 1 teaspoon dried thyme
- Salt and pepper to taste
- 1 lb boneless, skinless chicken breasts
- 1 cup frozen peas
- 1 bay leaf
- 2 cups shredded cooked chicken (from rotisserie chicken or leftovers)
- 2 tablespoons fresh parsley, chopped
- Lemon wedges, for serving (optional)

Instructions:

1. In a large pot, heat the olive oil over medium heat. Add the diced onion, carrots, and celery. Sauté for 5-7 minutes until vegetables are tender.

2. Add the minced garlic and cook for 1 minute until fragrant.

3. Pour in the chicken broth and add the bay leaf, dried thyme, salt, and pepper.

4. Add the raw chicken breasts to the pot and bring to a boil. Reduce heat to medium-low and simmer for 15-20 minutes until chicken is fully cooked through.

5. Remove the cooked chicken breasts from the pot and set aside to cool slightly.

6. Add the frozen peas to the pot and simmer for 5 minutes.

7. Shred or dice the cooked chicken breasts once cooled. Add the shredded chicken back to the pot.

8. Taste and adjust seasoning as needed with more salt, pepper or thyme if desired. Remove bay leaf. Stir in the fresh chopped parsley. Serve the chicken vegetable soup hot with a lemon wedge on the side if desired.

This recipe makes a classic, hearty chicken vegetable soup that's loaded with protein, nutrients and flavor. The fresh herbs add awesome aroma.

You can add other vegetables like diced potatoes, spinach or zucchini. For a creamy version, stir in some half-and-half at the end. Cooked pasta, barley or rice can also be added.

Top bowls with grated parmesan, oyster crackers or crusty bread for dipping. This hits the spot on a cold day! Leftovers also reheat well for easy lunches.

33. Turkey chili

Ingredients:
- 1 tablespoon olive oil
- 1 onion, diced
- 1 lb ground turkey
- 2 tablespoons chili powder
- 2 teaspoons ground cumin
- 1 teaspoon dried oregano
- 1/4 teaspoon cayenne pepper
 (optional for extra heat)
- 1 teaspoon salt
- 1/2 teaspoon black pepper
- 1 (15oz) can diced tomatoes with juices
- 1 (15oz) can tomato sauce
- 1 (15oz) can kidney beans, drained and rinsed
- 3 cloves garlic, minced
- 1 bell pepper, diced
- Toppings: shredded cheese, sour cream, sliced avocado, etc.

Instructions:

1. In a large pot or dutch oven, heat the olive oil over medium-high heat. Add the diced onion and cook for 2-3 minutes until translucent.

2. Add the garlic and cook for 1 minute until fragrant.

3. Add the ground turkey and cook for 5-7 minutes, breaking it up with a wooden spoon as it cooks, until no longer pink.

4. Stir in the chili powder, cumin, oregano, cayenne (if using), salt, and pepper. Cook for 2 more minutes.

5. Pour in the diced tomatoes with juices, tomato sauce, and kidney beans with their liquid. Add the diced bell pepper.

6. Bring the chili to a boil, then reduce heat and let it simmer for 20-25 minutes, until thickened and flavors have melded.

7. Taste and adjust seasoning as needed, adding more salt, pepper or chili powder to taste.

8. Serve the turkey chili hot with your favorite toppings like shredded cheese, sour cream, sliced avocado, green onions, tortilla chips, etc.

This turkey chili packs in all the classic, hearty flavors but uses lean ground turkey instead of beef for a healthier twist. The beans add protein and fiber too. You can use ground turkey breast or a blend of dark and light meat. Feel free to add extras like corn, diced zucchini or different types of beans.

Let the chili simmer for up to an hour if you have time - the flavors just get better! Serve with cornbread, tortilla chips or over rice. Leftovers also freeze beautifully for easy future meals.

34. Beef and vegetable stew

Ingredients:
- 1.5 lbs (680g) stewing beef, cut into bite-sized pieces
- 2 tablespoons olive oil
- 1 onion, chopped
- 3 cloves garlic, minced
- 4 carrots, peeled and sliced
- 3 potatoes, peeled and diced
- 2 stalks celery, sliced
- 1 can (14 oz/400g) diced tomatoes
- 4 cups (950ml) beef broth
- 1 teaspoon dried thyme
- 1 teaspoon dried rosemary
- Salt and pepper to taste
- Chopped fresh parsley for garnish (optional)

Instructions:

1. Heat olive oil in a large pot or Dutch oven over medium heat. Add the beef and cook until browned on all sides, about 5 minutes. Remove beef from the pot and set aside.

2. In the same pot, add a little more oil if needed, then add the onions and garlic. Cook until onions are softened, about 3-4 minutes.

3. Add carrots, potatoes, and celery to the pot. Cook for another 5 minutes, stirring occasionally.

4. Return the beef to the pot. Add diced tomatoes, beef broth, thyme, and rosemary. Season with salt and pepper to taste.

5. Bring the stew to a boil, then reduce the heat to low. Cover and simmer for 1.5 to 2 hours, or until the beef is tender and the vegetables are cooked through, stirring occasionally.

6. Once cooked, taste and adjust seasoning if necessary. Serve hot, garnished with chopped fresh parsley if desired.

Enjoy your hearty beef and vegetable stew!

35. White bean and kale soup

***Ingredients:**
- 2 tablespoons olive oil
- 1 onion, chopped
- 3 cloves garlic, minced
- 2 carrots, peeled and diced
- 2 stalks celery, diced
- 2 cans (15 oz/425g each) white beans (such as cannellini or navy beans), drained and rinsed
- 6 cups (1.4 liters) vegetable or chicken broth
- 1 bunch kale, stems removed and leaves chopped
- 1 teaspoon dried thyme
- 1 teaspoon dried rosemary
- Salt and pepper to taste
- Grated Parmesan cheese for serving (optional)

Instructions:

1. Heat olive oil in a large pot or Dutch oven over medium heat. Add the onion and cook until softened, about 3-4 minutes. Add the garlic and cook for another minute until fragrant.

2. Add carrots and celery to the pot. Cook for 5 minutes, stirring occasionally.

3. Stir in the white beans, vegetable or chicken broth, thyme, and rosemary. Bring the soup to a boil, then reduce the heat to low. Cover and simmer for 15-20 minutes, allowing the flavors to meld.

4. After simmering, use an immersion blender to partially blend the soup until it reaches your desired consistency. Alternatively, you can remove about 2 cups of the soup and blend it in a blender, then return it to the pot.

5. Add the chopped kale to the soup and simmer for an additional 5-10 minutes, or until the kale is tender.

6. Season with salt and pepper to taste. Serve hot, garnished with grated Parmesan cheese if desired.

This white bean and kale soup is hearty, nutritious, and perfect for a cozy meal. Enjoy!

36. Roasted red pepper and tomato soup

Ingredients:
- 4 large red bell peppers
- 2 tablespoons olive oil
- 1 onion, chopped
- 3 cloves garlic, minced
- 1 can (28 oz/800g) whole peeled tomatoes
- 4 cups (950ml) vegetable or chicken broth
- 1 teaspoon dried thyme
- 1 teaspoon dried basil
- Salt and pepper to taste
- 1/4 cup (60ml) heavy cream or coconut milk (optional)
- Fresh basil leaves for garnish (optional)

Instructions:

1. Preheat your oven to 400°F (200°C). Place the red bell peppers on a baking sheet lined with parchment paper. Roast them in the preheated oven for 20-25 minutes, or until the skins are charred and blistered, turning occasionally. Once roasted, remove the peppers from the oven and let them cool slightly. Once cooled, remove the skins, stems, and seeds, then chop the peppers into smaller pieces.

2. In a large pot or Dutch oven, heat olive oil over medium heat. Add the chopped onion and cook until softened, about 3-4 minutes. Add the minced garlic and cook for another minute until fragrant.

3. Add the roasted red peppers, canned tomatoes (with their juices), vegetable or chicken broth, dried thyme, and dried basil to the pot. Bring the mixture to a boil, then reduce the heat to low. Cover and simmer for 20-25 minutes to allow the flavors to meld.

4. Use an immersion blender to blend the soup until smooth. Alternatively, carefully transfer the soup to a blender and blend in batches until smooth.

5. Once blended, return the soup to the pot if necessary. Stir in the heavy cream or coconut milk, if using, to add creaminess to the soup. Season with salt and pepper to taste.

6. Serve hot, garnished with fresh basil leaves if desired.

Enjoy the rich flavors of this roasted red pepper and tomato soup!

37. Butternut squash soup

Ingredients:
- 1 medium-sized butternut squash (about 2 lbs/900g), peeled, seeded, and cubed
- 2 tablespoons olive oil
- 1 onion, chopped
- 2 cloves garlic, minced
- 1 carrot, peeled and chopped
- 1 celery stalk, chopped
- 4 cups (950ml) vegetable or chicken broth
- 1 teaspoon ground cinnamon
- 1/2 teaspoon ground nutmeg
- Salt and pepper to taste
- 1/2 cup (120ml) heavy cream or coconut milk (optional)
- Chopped fresh parsley or chives for garnish (optional)

Instructions:

1. In a large pot or Dutch oven, heat olive oil over medium heat. Add the chopped onion, garlic, carrot, and celery. Cook until the vegetables are softened, about 5-7 minutes.

2. Add the cubed butternut squash to the pot along with the vegetable or chicken broth, ground cinnamon, and ground nutmeg. Season with salt and pepper to taste.

3. Bring the mixture to a boil, then reduce the heat to low. Cover and simmer for 20-25 minutes, or until the butternut squash is tender.

4. Once the butternut squash is cooked, use an immersion blender to blend the soup until smooth. Alternatively, carefully transfer the soup to a blender and blend in batches until smooth.

5. Return the blended soup to the pot if necessary. Stir in the heavy cream or coconut milk, if using, to add creaminess to the soup.

6. Taste and adjust seasoning if needed. If the soup is too thick, you can thin it out with additional broth or water.

7. Serve hot, garnished with chopped fresh parsley or chives if desired.

Enjoy the creamy and comforting flavor of this butternut squash soup!

38. Lentil vegetable soup

Ingredients:
- 1 cup (200g) dried lentils, rinsed and drained
- 1 tablespoon olive oil
- 1 onion, chopped
- 2 carrots, peeled and diced
- 2 celery stalks, diced
- 3 cloves garlic, minced
- 1 can (14 oz/400g) diced tomatoes
- 6 cups (1.4 liters) vegetable or chicken broth
- 1 teaspoon ground cumin
- 1 teaspoon ground coriander
- 1/2 teaspoon smoked paprika
- Salt and pepper to taste
- 2 cups (about 200g) chopped vegetables (such as bell peppers, zucchini, or spinach)
- Juice of 1 lemon
- Chopped fresh parsley or cilantro for garnish (optional)

Instructions:
1. In a large pot or Dutch oven, heat olive oil over medium heat. Add the chopped onion, carrots, and celery. Cook until the vegetables are softened, about 5-7 minutes.

2. Add the minced garlic to the pot and cook for another minute until fragrant.

3. Stir in the rinsed lentils, diced tomatoes (with their juices), vegetable or chicken broth, ground cumin, ground coriander, and smoked paprika. Season with salt and pepper to taste.

4. Bring the soup to a boil, then reduce the heat to low. Cover and simmer for about 20-25 minutes, or until the lentils are tender.

5. Once the lentils are cooked, stir in the chopped vegetables of your choice. Cook for an additional 5-7 minutes, or until the vegetables are tender.

6. Remove the soup from heat and stir in the lemon juice. Taste and adjust seasoning if necessary.

7. Serve hot, garnished with chopped fresh parsley or cilantro if desired.

Enjoy the wholesome goodness of this lentil vegetable soup! It's even better the next day as the flavors meld together.

39. Shrimp and corn chowder

Ingredients:
- 1 lb (450g) shrimp, peeled and deveined
- 4 slices bacon, chopped
- 2 tablespoons butter
- 1 onion, chopped
- 2 cloves garlic, minced
- 2 potatoes, peeled and diced
- 2 cups (480ml) chicken broth
- 2 cups (480ml) milk
- 2 cups (about 340g) fresh or frozen corn kernels
- 1/2 teaspoon dried thyme
- 1/2 teaspoon Old Bay seasoning (optional)
- Salt and pepper to taste
- 1/4 cup (60ml) heavy cream (optional)
- Chopped fresh parsley or chives for garnish (optional)

Instructions:

1. In a large pot or Dutch oven, cook the chopped bacon over medium heat until crisp. Remove the bacon from the pot and set aside, leaving the bacon fat in the pot.

2. Add butter to the pot along with the chopped onion. Cook until the onion is softened, about 3-4 minutes. Add the minced garlic and cook for another minute until fragrant.

3. Stir in the diced potatoes, chicken broth, and milk. Bring the mixture to a simmer and cook until the potatoes are tender, about 10-12 minutes.

4. Once the potatoes are cooked, add the corn kernels, dried thyme, and Old Bay seasoning (if using) to the pot. Stir well and let it simmer for another 5 minutes.

5. Add the peeled and deveined shrimp to the pot and cook until they turn pink and opaque, about 3-4 minutes.

6. If desired, stir in the heavy cream to add extra creaminess to the chowder. Season with salt and pepper to taste.

7. Serve hot, garnished with the chopped cooked bacon, and fresh parsley or chives if desired.

Enjoy the rich and savory flavors of this shrimp and corn chowder!

40. Minestrone soup

Ingredients:
- 2 tablespoons olive oil
- 1 onion, chopped
- 2 cloves garlic, minced
- 2 carrots, diced
- 2 celery stalks, diced
- 1 zucchini, diced
- 1 yellow squash, diced
- 1 cup (150g) green beans, trimmed and cut into bite-sized pieces
- 1 can (14 oz/400g) diced tomatoes
- 6 cups (1.4 liters) vegetable or chicken broth
- 1 can (15 oz/425g) cannellini beans, drained and rinsed
- 1 cup (100g) small pasta (such as ditalini or small shells)
- 1 teaspoon dried oregano
- 1 teaspoon dried basil
- Salt and pepper to taste
- Grated Parmesan cheese for serving (optional)
- Chopped fresh parsley for garnish (optional)

Instructions:
1. In a large pot or Dutch oven, heat olive oil over medium heat. Add the chopped onion and cook until softened, about 3-4 minutes. Add the minced garlic and cook for another minute until fragrant.

2. Add the diced carrots, celery, zucchini, yellow squash, and green beans to the pot. Cook for about 5 minutes, stirring occasionally.

3. Stir in the diced tomatoes (with their juices) and vegetable or chicken broth. Bring the mixture to a boil, then reduce the heat to low. Cover and simmer for about 15 minutes, or until the vegetables are tender.

4. Add the cannellini beans and pasta to the pot. Cook for another 10-12 minutes, or until the pasta is al dente.

5. Stir in the dried oregano and basil. Season with salt and pepper to taste.

6. Serve hot, garnished with grated Parmesan cheese and chopped fresh parsley if desired.

Enjoy this comforting and flavorful minestrone soup! Serve it with crusty bread for a complete meal.

41. Quinoa salad with vegetables

Ingredients:
- 1 cup (170g) quinoa, rinsed
- 2 cups (480ml) water or vegetable broth
- 1 cup cherry tomatoes, halved
- 1 cucumber, diced
- 1 bell pepper, diced
- 1/4 cup (40g) red onion, finely chopped
- 1/4 cup (15g) fresh parsley, chopped
- 1/4 cup (15g) fresh cilantro, chopped (optional)
- Juice of 1-2 lemons
- 2 tablespoons extra virgin olive oil
- Salt and pepper to taste
- Optional additions: diced avocado, crumbled feta cheese, sliced olives, roasted chickpeas

Instructions:

1. In a medium saucepan, combine the quinoa and water or vegetable broth. Bring to a boil, then reduce the heat to low. Cover and simmer for 15-20 minutes, or until the quinoa is cooked and the liquid is absorbed. Remove from heat and let it cool slightly.

2. In a large mixing bowl, combine the cooked quinoa, cherry tomatoes, cucumber, bell pepper, red onion, parsley, and cilantro (if using).

3. In a small bowl, whisk together the lemon juice and extra virgin olive oil to make the dressing. Season with salt and pepper to taste.

4. Pour the dressing over the quinoa and vegetable mixture. Toss gently to combine, ensuring that the dressing coats all the ingredients evenly.

5. Taste and adjust seasoning if necessary. If desired, add optional additions such as diced avocado, crumbled feta cheese, sliced olives, or roasted chickpeas for extra flavor and texture.

6. Serve the quinoa salad immediately, or refrigerate it for at least 30 minutes to allow the flavors to meld together before serving.

Enjoy this refreshing and nutritious quinoa salad with vegetables as a light meal or side dish! It's perfect for picnics, potlucks, or as a healthy lunch option.

42. Roasted garlic parmesan cauliflower

Ingredients:
- 1 head of cauliflower, cut into florets
- 3 tablespoons olive oil
- 4 cloves garlic, minced
- 1/4 cup (25g) grated Parmesan cheese
- 1 teaspoon dried thyme
- 1/2 teaspoon paprika
- Salt and pepper to taste
- Chopped fresh parsley for garnish (optional)

Instructions:

1. Preheat your oven to 425°F (220°C). Line a baking sheet with parchment paper or aluminum foil for easy cleanup.

2. In a large mixing bowl, combine the cauliflower florets, olive oil, minced garlic, grated Parmesan cheese, dried thyme, paprika, salt, and pepper. Toss until the cauliflower is evenly coated with the seasoning mixture.

3. Spread the cauliflower florets in a single layer on the prepared baking sheet, making sure they are not overcrowded. This ensures even roasting.

4. Roast the cauliflower in the preheated oven for 25-30 minutes, or until the cauliflower is tender and golden brown, stirring halfway through to ensure even cooking.

5. Once the cauliflower is roasted to your desired level of crispiness, remove it from the oven.

6. Transfer the roasted garlic parmesan cauliflower to a serving dish and garnish with chopped fresh parsley, if desired.

7. Serve hot and enjoy as a flavorful side dish alongside your favorite main course.

This roasted garlic parmesan cauliflower is sure to be a hit at the dinner table. It's crispy, flavorful, and a perfect way to enjoy cauliflower in a new and delicious way.

43. Garlic green beans

Ingredients:
- 1 lb (450g) green beans, ends trimmed
- 2 tablespoons olive oil
- 4 cloves garlic, minced
- Salt and pepper to taste
- Red pepper flakes (optional)
- Lemon wedges for serving (optional)
- Grated Parmesan cheese for garnish (optional)
- Chopped fresh parsley for garnish (optional)

Instructions:

1. Bring a large pot of salted water to a boil. Add the green beans and cook for 2-3 minutes, or until they are bright green and crisp-tender. Be careful not to overcook them.

2. Drain the green beans and immediately transfer them to a bowl of ice water to stop the cooking process. This helps them retain their vibrant green color.

3. In a large skillet, heat the olive oil over medium heat. Add the minced garlic and cook for 1-2 minutes, or until fragrant. Be careful not to burn the garlic.

4. Add the blanched green beans to the skillet. Season with salt, pepper, and red pepper flakes (if using). Toss well to coat the green beans evenly with the garlic-infused oil.

5. Cook the green beans for 2-3 minutes, stirring occasionally, until they are heated through and slightly tender.

6. Remove the skillet from the heat and transfer the garlic green beans to a serving dish.

7. Garnish with grated Parmesan cheese and chopped fresh parsley, if desired. Serve hot with lemon wedges on the side for squeezing over the green beans.

Enjoy these flavorful garlic green beans as a tasty side dish with your favorite meals!

44. Wild rice pilaf

Ingredients:
- 1 cup (180g) wild rice
- 2 cups (480ml) vegetable or chicken broth
- 1 tablespoon olive oil or butter
- 1 onion, finely chopped
- 2 cloves garlic, minced
- 1 carrot, diced
- 1 celery stalk, diced
- 1/4 cup (30g) sliced almonds
- 1/4 cup (30g) dried cranberries or raisins
- 1/4 teaspoon dried thyme
- Salt and pepper to taste
- Chopped fresh parsley for garnish (optional)

Instructions:
1. Rinse the wild rice under cold water in a fine-mesh sieve or strainer.

2. In a medium saucepan, combine the rinsed wild rice and vegetable or chicken broth. Bring to a boil, then reduce the heat to low. Cover and simmer for 40-45 minutes, or until the wild rice is tender and most of the liquid is absorbed. Remove from heat and let it sit, covered, for 5 minutes.

3. While the wild rice is cooking, heat the olive oil or butter in a large skillet over medium heat. Add the chopped onion, minced garlic, diced carrot, and diced celery. Cook until the vegetables are softened, about 5-7 minutes.

4. Stir in the sliced almonds and dried cranberries or raisins. Cook for another 2-3 minutes, or until the almonds are lightly toasted and the cranberries or raisins are softened.

5. Once the wild rice is cooked, fluff it with a fork and transfer it to the skillet with the cooked vegetables, almonds, and cranberries or raisins. Stir well to combine.

6. Season the wild rice pilaf with dried thyme, salt, and pepper to taste. Adjust seasoning if necessary.

7. Transfer the wild rice pilaf to a serving dish and garnish with chopped fresh parsley, if desired.

Enjoy this delicious wild rice pilaf as a flavorful and nutritious side dish alongside your favorite main courses!

45. Roasted root vegetables

Ingredients:
- 2 lbs (about 900g) mixed root vegetables (such as carrots, parsnips, sweet potatoes, potatoes, turnips, and beets), peeled and cut into bite-sized pieces
- 3 tablespoons olive oil
- 2 cloves garlic, minced
- 1 teaspoon dried thyme
- 1 teaspoon dried rosemary
- Salt and pepper to taste
- Chopped fresh parsley for garnish (optional)

Instructions:

1. Preheat your oven to 425°F (220°C). Line a large baking sheet with parchment paper or aluminum foil for easy cleanup.

2. In a large mixing bowl, combine the bite-sized root vegetables with olive oil, minced garlic, dried thyme, dried rosemary, salt, and pepper. Toss well to coat the vegetables evenly with the seasoning mixture.

3. Spread the seasoned root vegetables in a single layer on the prepared baking sheet, making sure they are not overcrowded. This ensures even roasting and caramelization.

4. Roast the root vegetables in the preheated oven for 25-30 minutes, or until they are tender and golden brown, stirring halfway through to ensure even cooking.

5. Once the root vegetables are roasted to your desired level of crispiness, remove them from the oven.

6. Transfer the roasted root vegetables to a serving dish and garnish with chopped fresh parsley, if desired.

7. Serve hot and enjoy these flavorful roasted root vegetables as a delicious side dish alongside your favorite main courses.

Feel free to customize this recipe by adding your favorite herbs and spices or experimenting with different combinations of root vegetables. It's a versatile dish that's sure to be a hit at the dinner table!

46. Cucumber tomato salad

Ingredients:
- 2 large cucumbers, sliced
- 2 large tomatoes, diced
- 1/4 cup (60ml) red onion, thinly sliced
- 2 tablespoons fresh parsley, chopped
- 2 tablespoons fresh basil, chopped
- 2 tablespoons extra virgin olive oil
- 1 tablespoon red wine vinegar or balsamic vinegar
- Salt and pepper to taste
- Optional: crumbled feta cheese, sliced olives, chopped fresh mint

Instructions:

1. In a large mixing bowl, combine the sliced cucumbers, diced tomatoes, sliced red onion, chopped parsley, and chopped basil.

2. In a small bowl, whisk together the extra virgin olive oil and red wine vinegar or balsamic vinegar to make the dressing.

3. Pour the dressing over the cucumber and tomato mixture. Toss gently to coat all the ingredients evenly with the dressing.

4. Season the salad with salt and pepper to taste. Adjust seasoning if necessary.

5. If desired, add optional ingredients such as crumbled feta cheese, sliced olives, or chopped fresh mint for extra flavor and texture.

6. Serve the cucumber tomato salad immediately, or refrigerate it for at least 30 minutes to allow the flavors to meld together before serving.

This cucumber tomato salad is light, refreshing, and bursting with fresh flavors. It's a perfect side dish for grilled meats, fish, or as a standalone dish for a light lunch or dinner. Enjoy!

47. Mashed sweet potatoes

Ingredients:
- 2 lbs (about 900g) sweet potatoes, peeled and diced
- 4 tablespoons unsalted butter
- 1/4 cup (60ml) milk or cream
- 2 tablespoons maple syrup or honey (optional)
- 1/2 teaspoon ground cinnamon
- 1/4 teaspoon ground nutmeg
- Salt to taste
- Chopped fresh parsley or chives for garnish (optional)

Instructions:

1. Place the diced sweet potatoes in a large pot and cover them with cold water. Bring the water to a boil over high heat, then reduce the heat to medium and simmer the sweet potatoes for 15-20 minutes, or until they are fork-tender.

2. Once the sweet potatoes are cooked, drain them thoroughly and return them to the pot.

3. Add the unsalted butter to the pot with the cooked sweet potatoes. Mash the sweet potatoes and butter together using a potato masher or fork until they reach your desired consistency.

4. Gradually add the milk or cream to the mashed sweet potatoes, stirring until the mixture is smooth and creamy. Add more milk or cream as needed to achieve the desired consistency.

5. If using, stir in the maple syrup or honey, ground cinnamon, ground nutmeg, and salt to taste. Adjust seasoning according to your preference.

6. Transfer the mashed sweet potatoes to a serving dish and garnish with chopped fresh parsley or chives, if desired.

7. Serve hot and enjoy these creamy and flavorful mashed sweet potatoes as a delicious side dish for any meal.

These mashed sweet potatoes are perfect for Thanksgiving, Christmas, or any time you're craving a comforting and nutritious side dish. Enjoy!

48. Sauteed kale with garlic

Ingredients:
- 1 bunch kale
- 2 tablespoons olive oil
- 3 cloves garlic, minced
- Salt and pepper to taste
- Red pepper flakes (optional)
- Lemon wedges for serving (optional)

Instructions:

1. Wash the kale thoroughly under cold water and remove the tough stems. Tear or chop the kale leaves into bite-sized pieces.

2. Heat the olive oil in a large skillet over medium heat. Add the minced garlic and sauté for about 1 minute, or until fragrant. Be careful not to let the garlic burn.

3. Add the chopped kale leaves to the skillet in batches, allowing each batch to wilt slightly before adding more. Use tongs to toss the kale leaves with the garlic and olive oil.

4. Continue to sauté the kale until it is wilted and tender, about 5-7 minutes. Stir occasionally to ensure even cooking.

5. Season the sautéed kale with salt, pepper, and red pepper flakes (if using), to taste. Adjust seasoning according to your preference.

6. Once the kale is cooked to your liking, remove the skillet from the heat.

7. Serve the sautéed kale hot, with lemon wedges on the side for squeezing over the kale if desired.

Enjoy this flavorful and nutritious sautéed kale with garlic as a tasty side dish with your favorite main courses! It's quick and easy to make and packed with healthy greens.

49. Baked acorn squash

Ingredients:
- 2 acorn squash
- 2 tablespoons olive oil or melted butter
- 2 tablespoons brown sugar or maple syrup
- Salt and pepper to taste
- Optional: cinnamon, nutmeg, or other spices of your choice

Instructions:

1. Preheat your oven to 400°F (200°C). Line a baking sheet with parchment paper or aluminum foil for easy cleanup.

2. Cut each acorn squash in half lengthwise and scoop out the seeds and stringy pulp using a spoon. You can save the seeds for roasting if you like.

3. Place the acorn squash halves cut-side up on the prepared baking sheet.

4. Brush the cut sides of the squash halves with olive oil or melted butter. Sprinkle each half with brown sugar or drizzle with maple syrup. Season with salt and pepper to taste.

5. If desired, sprinkle the squash halves with cinnamon, nutmeg, or other spices of your choice for extra flavor.

6. Place the baking sheet in the preheated oven and bake the squash for 40-50 minutes, or until the flesh is fork-tender and caramelized around the edges.

7. Once the squash is baked, remove it from the oven and let it cool for a few minutes before serving.

8. Serve the baked acorn squash halves hot, as a delicious side dish for your favorite autumn meals.

Enjoy the natural sweetness and buttery texture of baked acorn squash! It's a comforting and nutritious addition to any dinner table.

50. Black bean and corn salad

Ingredients:
- 1 can (15 oz/425g) black beans, drained and rinsed
- 1 cup (150g) corn kernels (fresh, canned, or thawed if frozen)
- 1 bell pepper (red, yellow, or orange), diced
- 1/2 red onion, finely chopped
- 1 jalapeño pepper, seeded and minced (optional, for some heat)
- 1/4 cup (15g) fresh cilantro, chopped
- Juice of 1-2 limes
- 2 tablespoons extra virgin olive oil
- 1 teaspoon ground cumin
- 1/2 teaspoon chili powder
- Salt and pepper to taste
- Avocado slices for garnish (optional)

Instructions:

1. In a large mixing bowl, combine the black beans, corn kernels, diced bell pepper, finely chopped red onion, minced jalapeño pepper (if using), and chopped fresh cilantro.

2. In a small bowl, whisk together the lime juice, extra virgin olive oil, ground cumin, chili powder, salt, and pepper to make the dressing.

3. Pour the dressing over the black bean and corn mixture. Toss gently to coat all the ingredients evenly with the dressing.

4. Taste the salad and adjust seasoning if necessary. Add more lime juice, salt, or pepper according to your preference.

5. Cover the bowl and refrigerate the black bean and corn salad for at least 30 minutes to allow the flavors to meld together before serving.

6. Just before serving, garnish the salad with avocado slices, if desired.

7. Serve chilled or at room temperature as a delicious side dish or light meal.

Enjoy this flavorful and colorful black bean and corn salad! It's packed with protein, fiber, and vitamins, making it a healthy and satisfying dish for any occasion.

51. Green tea

Ingredients:
- 1 teaspoon green tea leaves (or 1 tea bag)
- Hot water (not boiling, around 160-180°F or 70-80°C)
- Optional: honey, lemon, mint leaves, or other flavorings

Instructions:

1. Boil water and then let it cool for a few minutes to reach the ideal temperature for green tea (around 160-180°F or 70-80°C). Water that is too hot can make the tea taste bitter.

2. Place the green tea leaves in a teapot or a cup. If using tea bags, place one tea bag in a cup.

3. Pour the hot water over the tea leaves or tea bag.

4. Steep the tea for about 2-3 minutes. Steeping time can vary depending on personal preference and the specific type of green tea you're using. Some green teas may require shorter or longer steeping times.

5. Once the tea has steeped to your desired strength, remove the tea leaves or tea bag.

6. If desired, you can sweeten your green tea with honey or add a squeeze of lemon for extra flavor. You can also add mint leaves or other herbs for a refreshing twist.

7. Serve your green tea hot and enjoy!

Green tea is not only delicious but also known for its health benefits, including being rich in antioxidants and potentially offering various protective effects for the body. So, savor your cup of green tea and reap its many benefits!

52. Herbal teas (e.g. ginger, peppermint)

Ingredients:
- 1-inch piece of fresh ginger root, thinly sliced or grated
- 1-2 cups (240-480ml) water
- Optional: honey, lemon slices

Instructions:
1. Place the thinly sliced or grated ginger root in a microwave-safe mug. Pour 1-2 cups of water over the ginger slices in the mug.

2. Microwave the mug on high for 2-3 minutes, or until the water comes to a boil. Let the ginger steep in the hot water for 3-5 minutes, depending on how strong you like your tea.

3. Once steeped, strain out the ginger slices or leave them in the tea for extra flavor.

4. If desired, add honey and/or lemon slices to sweeten and flavor your ginger tea. Stir well and enjoy your soothing ginger tea!

Peppermint Tea:
Ingredients:
- 1-2 teaspoons dried peppermint leaves or 1-2 peppermint tea bags
- 1-2 cups (240-480ml) water
- Optional: honey, lemon slices

Instructions:
1. Place the dried peppermint leaves or peppermint tea bag in a microwave-safe mug.

2. Pour 1-2 cups of water over the peppermint leaves or tea bag in the mug.

3. Microwave the mug on high for 2-3 minutes, or until the water comes to a boil.

4. Let the peppermint steep in the hot water for 3-5 minutes, depending on how strong you like your tea. Once steeped, remove the peppermint leaves or tea bag from the mug.

5. If desired, add honey and/or lemon slices to sweeten and flavor your peppermint tea. Stir well and enjoy your refreshing peppermint tea!

Remember to use caution when handling hot liquids and always use microwave-safe containers. These herbal teas are not only delicious but also offer potential health benefits and can be enjoyed at any time of the day.

53. Fruit-infused water

Ingredients:
- Fresh fruits of your choice (such as berries, citrus fruits, melons, pineapple, cucumber, etc.)
- Fresh herbs or spices (optional, such as mint, basil, ginger, cinnamon, etc.)
- Water
- Ice cubes (optional)

Instructions:
1. Wash and prepare your fruits by slicing, chopping, or mashing them, depending on your preference. Remove any seeds or pits from fruits like berries or citrus fruits.

2. Place the prepared fruits and herbs or spices in a large pitcher or jar.

3. Fill the pitcher or jar with water. You can use still or sparkling water, depending on your preference.

4. Stir the ingredients gently to combine.

5. Refrigerate the fruit-infused water for at least 1-2 hours to allow the flavors to infuse into the water. For a stronger flavor, you can refrigerate the water overnight.

6. Once chilled, you can strain out the fruits and herbs if desired, or leave them in the water for extra flavor.

7. Serve the fruit-infused water over ice cubes if desired, and enjoy!

Here are a few fruit-infused water combinations to try:

- Citrus Mint: Slices of lemon, lime, and orange with fresh mint leaves.
- Berry Blast: Mixed berries such as strawberries, blueberries, and raspberries.
- Tropical Paradise: Pineapple chunks, mango slices, and coconut water.
- Cucumber Lemon: Slices of cucumber and lemon with a sprig of fresh basil.
- Watermelon Basil: Cubes of watermelon with fresh basil leaves.

Feel free to get creative and experiment with different fruit and herb combinations to create your own custom fruit-infused water recipes. It's a delicious and healthy way to stay hydrated and enjoy the natural flavors of fruits and herbs.

54. Vegetable juices

Ingredients:
- Assorted vegetables of your choice (such as carrots, celery, cucumber, kale, spinach, beets, bell peppers, etc.)
- Optional: lemon or lime for added flavor

Instructions:
1. Wash and prepare your vegetables by cutting them into smaller pieces that will fit into your juicer chute.

2. Feed the vegetables through your juicer, one at a time, until you have extracted the desired amount of juice.

3. If using, squeeze in some lemon or lime juice for added flavor. You can also add a small piece of ginger or a handful of fresh herbs like parsley or cilantro for extra taste.

4. Stir the juice well to combine any added flavors.

5. Serve the vegetable juice immediately over ice if desired, or refrigerate it for later consumption.

Tips:
- Experiment with different vegetable combinations to find the flavors you enjoy the most. Carrots, apples, and ginger are a classic combination that's both sweet and spicy.
- Use fresh, organic vegetables whenever possible to maximize the nutrient content of your juice.
- Drink your vegetable juice soon after making it to ensure you get the most nutrients. Fresh juice can oxidize quickly, which may reduce its nutritional value.
- If you don't have a juicer, you can make vegetable juice using a blender and then strain the mixture through a fine-mesh sieve or cheesecloth to remove the pulp.
- Don't be afraid to get creative! Vegetable juice is a versatile beverage, and you can customize it to suit your taste preferences and nutritional needs.

By incorporating homemade vegetable juices into your diet, you can boost your intake of vitamins, minerals, and antioxidants while enjoying delicious and refreshing beverages.

55. Almond milk smoothies

Ingredients:
- 1 cup unsweetened almond milk
- 1 ripe banana, frozen
- 1/2 cup frozen berries (such as strawberries, blueberries, or raspberries)
- 1 tablespoon almond butter or peanut butter (optional)
- 1 tablespoon honey, maple syrup, or other sweetener (optional)
- Ice cubes (optional, for a thicker smoothie)

Instructions:

1. In a blender, combine the unsweetened almond milk, frozen banana, frozen berries, almond butter or peanut butter (if using), and sweetener (if using).

2. Blend the ingredients on high speed until smooth and creamy. If the smoothie is too thick, you can add more almond milk to reach your desired consistency.

3. Taste the smoothie and adjust the sweetness if necessary by adding more honey, maple syrup, or other sweetener.

4. If you prefer a colder smoothie, you can add a few ice cubes to the blender and blend until smooth.

5. Once blended to your liking, pour the smoothie into glasses and serve immediately.

Variations:

- Green Smoothie: Add a handful of fresh spinach or kale to the basic recipe for an extra boost of nutrients.
- Chocolate Almond Smoothie: Add a tablespoon of cocoa powder or chocolate protein powder to the basic recipe for a rich and indulgent treat.
- Tropical Almond Smoothie: Use frozen pineapple, mango, and banana instead of berries for a taste of the tropics.
- Nutty Almond Smoothie: Add a tablespoon of chopped nuts (such as almonds, walnuts, or pecans) to the basic recipe for added crunch and flavor.

Feel free to customize your almond milk smoothies with your favorite fruits, vegetables, and flavorings to create delicious and nutritious beverages that you'll love to enjoy any time of day.

56. Golden milk (turmeric milk)

Ingredients:
- 2 cups milk (dairy or plant-based, such as almond milk, coconut milk, or cashew milk)
- 1 teaspoon ground turmeric
- 1/2 teaspoon ground cinnamon
- 1/4 teaspoon ground ginger
- Pinch of ground black pepper (helps with the absorption of turmeric)
- Sweetener of your choice, such as honey, maple syrup, or agave syrup, to taste
- Optional: 1 teaspoon coconut oil or ghee (clarified butter)

Instructions:

1. In a small saucepan, heat the milk over medium-low heat until it is warm but not boiling.

2. Add the ground turmeric, ground cinnamon, ground ginger, and pinch of black pepper to the warm milk. Stir well to combine.

3. If using, add the coconut oil or ghee to the milk mixture. This adds richness and can enhance the absorption of turmeric.

4. Continue to heat the milk mixture over low heat, stirring occasionally, for about 5 minutes. Be careful not to let it come to a boil.

5. Once the golden milk is heated through and well-combined, remove it from the heat.

6. Taste the golden milk and sweeten it with your preferred sweetener, adjusting to your taste preferences.

7. Pour the golden milk into mugs and serve warm.

Golden milk can be enjoyed as a comforting beverage any time of day, but it's particularly soothing in the evening before bedtime. The warm spices and creamy texture make it a cozy treat that's also packed with potential health benefits.

57. Coconut water

Fresh Coconut Water:

1. Select a fresh coconut that feels heavy for its size and has no visible cracks.
2. Use a sharp knife to carefully cut off the top of the coconut, exposing the inner flesh.
3. Pour the coconut water into a glass or drink it straight from the coconut using a straw.
4. Enjoy the fresh, natural flavor of coconut water as a refreshing beverage.

Packaged Coconut Water:

1. Purchase packaged coconut water from a grocery store or health food store. Look for options that contain no added sugars or artificial ingredients.
2. Chill the coconut water in the refrigerator for a refreshing and cold beverage.
3. Pour the coconut water into a glass over ice, if desired, or drink it straight from the bottle or carton.
4. Enjoy the convenient and hydrating benefits of packaged coconut water on the go or at home.

Coconut Water Smoothie:

1. Combine coconut water with your favorite fruits, such as berries, bananas, or mangoes, in a blender.
2. Add a handful of leafy greens, like spinach or kale, for added nutrition.
3. Blend until smooth and creamy.
4. Pour the coconut water smoothie into a glass and enjoy as a nutritious and hydrating snack or breakfast option.

Coconut Water Cocktail:

1. Mix coconut water with your favorite spirits, such as rum or vodka, for a refreshing cocktail.
2. Add a splash of citrus juice, like lime or pineapple, for extra flavor.
3. Serve the coconut water cocktail over ice in a glass with a garnish of fresh fruit or herbs.
4. Enjoy the tropical flavors of a coconut water cocktail as a refreshing drink for parties or gatherings.

Whether enjoyed fresh from a coconut or packaged from the store, coconut water is a delicious and hydrating beverage that's perfect for staying refreshed and replenished throughout the day.

58. Unsweetened coffee

Ingredients:
- Freshly ground coffee beans
- Water

Instructions:

1. Start by grinding your coffee beans to a medium-coarse consistency. The grind size will depend on your brewing method. For example, use a coarser grind for French press and a finer grind for espresso.

2. Measure out the desired amount of coffee grounds based on your preferred strength. A standard ratio is about 1-2 tablespoons of coffee grounds for every 6 ounces of water, but you can adjust this to suit your taste.

3. Heat water to the appropriate temperature for your brewing method. For most methods, water should be between 195°F to 205°F (90°C to 96°C).

4. Place the coffee grounds in your brewing device (such as a drip coffee maker, French press, pour-over cone, or espresso machine).

5. Pour the hot water over the coffee grounds, making sure to saturate them evenly.

6. Allow the coffee to brew for the appropriate amount of time. This can vary depending on your brewing method and personal preference. Typically, brewing times range from 3-5 minutes for methods like pour-over or French press, and 25-30 seconds for espresso.

7. Once the coffee has finished brewing, carefully remove the grounds or filter, and pour the brewed coffee into your mug.

8. Let the coffee cool for a minute or two before enjoying it, as it may be very hot.

9. Taste the coffee and adjust as necessary. If you prefer your coffee stronger, you can use more coffee grounds next time. If you find it too strong, you can dilute it with hot water.

10. Serve your unsweetened coffee black, or add milk or cream if desired.

With these simple steps, you can enjoy a delicious cup of unsweetened coffee tailored to your taste preferences and brewing method.

59. Chia seed drinks

Basic Chia Seed Drink:
Ingredients:
- 2 cups water or your choice of liquid (such as coconut water, fruit juice, almond milk, etc.)
- 2 tablespoons chia seeds
- Sweetener of your choice, such as honey, maple syrup, or agave syrup (optional)
- Flavorings of your choice, such as lemon or lime juice, vanilla extract, or fruit puree (optional)
- Ice cubes (optional)

Instructions:

1. In a glass or jar, combine the water or liquid of your choice with the chia seeds.

2. Stir the mixture well to evenly distribute the chia seeds.

3. Let the mixture sit for about 5-10 minutes, stirring occasionally. This allows the chia seeds to absorb the liquid and form a gel-like consistency.

4. If using, add sweetener and flavorings to the chia seed mixture, adjusting to your taste preferences.

5. If desired, add ice cubes to the drink to chill it.

6. Stir the chia seed drink again before serving to ensure that the seeds are evenly distributed throughout the liquid. Serve the chia seed drink cold and enjoy!

Variations:
- Fruity Chia Seed Drink: Add fruit juice or puree, such as orange juice, pineapple juice, or berry puree, to the chia seed mixture for a fruity twist.

- Creamy Chia Seed Drink: Use almond milk, coconut milk, or another creamy liquid as the base for your chia seed drink. Add a splash of vanilla extract for extra flavor.

- Citrus Chia Seed Drink: Squeeze fresh lemon or lime juice into the chia seed mixture for a tangy and refreshing drink.

Feel free to experiment with different flavor combinations and ingredients to create your own custom chia seed drinks. They're a nutritious and hydrating beverage option that's perfect for any time of day!

60. Green smoothies

Ingredients:
- 1 cup leafy greens (such as spinach, kale, or Swiss chard)
- 1 ripe banana, fresh or frozen
- 1/2 cup fresh or frozen fruit (such as berries, mango, pineapple, or apple)
- 1/2 cup liquid (such as water, coconut water, almond milk, or Greek yogurt)
- Optional: 1 tablespoon nut butter (such as almond butter or peanut butter) for added creaminess and protein
- Optional: 1 tablespoon chia seeds or flaxseeds for added fiber and omega-3 fatty acids
- Ice cubes (optional, for a colder smoothie)

Instructions:

1. Place the leafy greens, banana, fruit, liquid, nut butter, and seeds (if using) in a blender.

2. Blend the ingredients on high speed until smooth and creamy. If the smoothie is too thick, you can add more liquid to reach your desired consistency.

3. Taste the smoothie and adjust the sweetness if necessary by adding more fruit or a natural sweetener like honey or maple syrup.

4. If using, add ice cubes to the blender and blend until smooth for a colder smoothie.

5. Once blended to your liking, pour the green smoothie into glasses and serve immediately.

Variations:
- Tropical Green Smoothie: Use mango, pineapple, and coconut water for a taste of the tropics.
- Berry Green Smoothie: Use a combination of berries such as strawberries, blueberries, and raspberries for a colorful and antioxidant-rich smoothie.
- Citrus Green Smoothie: Add orange or grapefruit segments along with a splash of orange juice for a zesty and refreshing smoothie.
- Protein Green Smoothie: Add a scoop of protein powder or Greek yogurt for an extra protein boost.
- Green Detox Smoothie: Add cucumber, celery, and parsley or cilantro for a detoxifying and cleansing smoothie.

Feel free to customize your green smoothies with your favorite fruits, vegetables, and flavorings to create delicious and nutritious beverages that you'll love to enjoy any time of day.

61. Hummus with veggie sticks

Ingredients:
For the hummus:
- 1 can (15 ounces) chickpeas (also known as garbanzo beans), drained and rinsed
- 2 cloves garlic, minced
- 3 tablespoons tahini (sesame seed paste)
- 2 tablespoons fresh lemon juice
- 2 tablespoons extra virgin olive oil
- 1/2 teaspoon ground cumin
- Salt and pepper to taste
- Water (as needed to adjust consistency)

For the veggie sticks: Assorted vegetables such as carrots, cucumber, bell peppers, celery, and cherry tomatoes, washed and cut into sticks

Instructions:
For the hummus:
1. In a food processor or blender, combine the drained chickpeas, minced garlic, tahini, lemon juice, olive oil, ground cumin, salt, and pepper.

2. Blend the ingredients until smooth and creamy. If the hummus is too thick, you can add water, a tablespoon at a time, until you reach your desired consistency.

3. Taste the hummus and adjust the seasoning if necessary, adding more salt, pepper, or lemon juice to taste.

4. Once the hummus is ready, transfer it to a serving bowl and drizzle with a little extra olive oil, if desired. You can also sprinkle with a pinch of paprika or chopped fresh herbs for garnish.

For the veggie sticks:
1. Wash and prepare your assortment of vegetables by cutting them into sticks. Arrange the veggie sticks on a serving platter or plate alongside the bowl of hummus. Serve the hummus with the veggie sticks for dipping.

Tips:
- You can customize your hummus by adding additional ingredients such as roasted red peppers, sun-dried tomatoes, or fresh herbs like parsley or cilantro.
- For an extra flavor boost, try sprinkling the hummus with a pinch of smoked paprika, za'atar seasoning, or toasted sesame seeds.
- Hummus and veggie sticks make a great addition to party platters or picnics, and they're also perfect for a healthy snack any time of day.

62. Greek yogurt with berries

Ingredients:
- 1 cup Greek yogurt (plain or flavored)
- Assorted berries (such as strawberries, blueberries, raspberries, blackberries)
- Optional: honey or maple syrup for sweetness
- Optional: granola or nuts for added crunch

Instructions:

1. Spoon the Greek yogurt into a serving bowl or individual serving cups.

2. Wash the berries thoroughly and slice any larger berries, if desired.

3. Arrange the berries on top of the Greek yogurt.

4. If desired, drizzle honey or maple syrup over the yogurt and berries for added sweetness.

5. Optionally, sprinkle granola or nuts over the yogurt and berries for extra texture and flavor.

6. Serve the Greek yogurt with berries immediately and enjoy!

Variations:

- Frozen Yogurt and Berry Parfait* Use frozen Greek yogurt instead of fresh, and layer it in a glass with alternating layers of berries for a refreshing parfait.

- Smoothie Bowl: Blend Greek yogurt with your favorite berries and a splash of liquid (such as milk or juice) until smooth. Pour the mixture into a bowl and top with additional berries, granola, and nuts for a nutritious smoothie bowl.

- Yogurt Bark: Spread Greek yogurt onto a baking sheet lined with parchment paper. Sprinkle berries over the yogurt and freeze until firm. Break the yogurt bark into pieces and enjoy as a healthy and refreshing snack.

Greek yogurt with berries is versatile, customizable, and perfect for any time of day. It's a satisfying and nutritious option that's sure to become a favorite!

63. Guacamole with baked tortilla chips

-3 ripe avocados
- 1 small red onion, finely diced
- 2 tomatoes, diced
- 1 jalapeño pepper, seeded and minced (optional)
- 1/4 cup chopped fresh cilantro
- Juice of 1 lime
- Salt and pepper to taste

Baked Tortilla Chips Ingredients:
- 6 small corn tortillas
- Cooking spray
- Salt to taste

Guacamole Instructions:
1. Cut the avocados in half, remove the pits, and scoop the flesh into a mixing bowl.

2. Mash the avocado with a fork until smooth or until you reach your desired consistency.

3. Add the diced red onion, diced tomatoes, minced jalapeño (if using), chopped cilantro, lime juice, salt, and pepper to the mashed avocado. Mix until well combined.

4. Taste and adjust seasoning if necessary. Add more lime juice or salt according to your preference.

5. Cover the guacamole with plastic wrap, making sure the wrap is directly touching the surface to prevent browning. Refrigerate until ready to serve.

Baked Tortilla Chips Instructions:
1. Preheat your oven to 350°F (175°C).

2. Stack the corn tortillas and cut them into wedges using a sharp knife or a pizza cutter. Arrange the tortilla wedges in a single layer on a baking sheet lined with parchment paper.

3. Lightly spray the tortilla wedges with cooking spray and sprinkle with salt. Bake in the preheated oven for 10-12 minutes, or until the chips are golden brown and crispy.

4. Remove the baking sheet from the oven and let the tortilla chips cool slightly before serving.

Serve the guacamole with the baked tortilla chips on the side. Enjoy your homemade guacamole and baked tortilla chips as a delicious and healthy snack or appetizer!

Feel free to customize the guacamole by adding additional ingredients such as diced garlic, chopped green onions, or diced bell peppers. You can also adjust the spiciness by leaving the jalapeño seeds in or omitting it altogether. Enjoy!

64. Hard boiled eggs

Ingredients: Eggs (as many as desired)

Instructions:
1. Place the eggs in a single layer in a saucepan or pot. Make sure the eggs are not stacked on top of each other.

2. Add enough water to the pot to cover the eggs by about an inch.

3. Place the pot on the stove and bring the water to a boil over medium-high heat.

4. Once the water comes to a rolling boil, remove the pot from the heat and cover it with a lid.

5. Let the eggs sit in the hot water, covered, for about 9-12 minutes, depending on the size of the eggs and how well-done you want them. 9 minutes for softer yolks, 12 minutes for firmer yolks.

6. While the eggs are cooking, prepare a bowl of ice water.

7. After the eggs have cooked for the desired amount of time, use a slotted spoon to transfer them to the bowl of ice water to cool down quickly. This helps stop the cooking process and makes the eggs easier to peel.

8. Let the eggs sit in the ice water bath for about 5 minutes to cool completely.

9. Once the eggs are cool, remove them from the water and gently tap each egg on a hard surface to crack the shell. Roll the egg between your hands to loosen the shell, then peel it off starting from the larger end, where the air pocket is located.

10. Rinse the peeled eggs under cold water to remove any bits of shell, if necessary.

11. The hard-boiled eggs are now ready to be enjoyed immediately or stored in the refrigerator for later use.

Hard-boiled eggs are a nutritious and convenient snack, perfect for adding protein to salads, sandwiches, or as a simple on-the-go snack.

65. Apple with almond butter

Ingredients:
- 1 apple (any variety you prefer)
- Almond butter (or your favorite nut butter)

Instructions:

1. Wash the apple thoroughly under running water and pat it dry with a clean towel.

2. Core the apple and slice it into wedges or rounds, depending on your preference. You can leave the skin on for added fiber and nutrients, or peel it off if you prefer.

3. Spread a generous amount of almond butter onto each apple slice. You can use store-bought almond butter or make your own at home.

4. Arrange the almond butter-covered apple slices on a plate or serving tray.. Serve immediately and enjoy your delicious and nutritious snack!

Variations:

- Toppings: Sprinkle the almond butter-covered apple slices with toppings such as cinnamon, chopped nuts, or granola for added flavor and texture.

- Dipping: Instead of spreading almond butter directly onto the apple slices, serve the almond butter in a small bowl on the side for dipping.

- Sandwiches: Make apple and almond butter sandwiches by spreading almond butter between two apple slices to create a tasty and portable snack.

- Additions: Enhance your apple and almond butter snack by adding additional toppings like sliced bananas, raisins, or shredded coconut.

Apple with almond butter is a satisfying and wholesome snack that's perfect for any time of day. It provides a good balance of carbohydrates, healthy fats, and fiber to keep you feeling full and energized.

66. Edamame

Ingredients: Edamame pods (fresh or frozen)

Instructions:
Boiling Method:
1. Bring a pot of water to a boil over high heat.
2. Add the edamame pods to the boiling water.
3. Boil the edamame pods for about 3-5 minutes, or until they are tender.
4. Once cooked, drain the edamame pods and rinse them under cold water to stop the cooking process.
5. Season the edamame pods with salt or other seasonings of your choice, if desired.
6. Serve the edamame pods warm or chilled and enjoy by squeezing the beans out of the pods directly into your mouth.

Steaming Method:

1. Place the edamame pods in a steamer basket.
2. Steam the edamame pods for about 5-7 minutes, or until they are tender.
3. Once cooked, remove the edamame pods from the steamer basket.
4. Season the edamame pods with salt or other seasonings of your choice, if desired.
5. Serve the edamame pods warm or chilled and enjoy by squeezing the beans out of the pods directly into your mouth.

Microwaving Method:
1. Place the edamame pods in a microwave-safe dish.
2. Add a small amount of water to the dish.
3. Cover the dish with a microwave-safe lid or microwave-safe plastic wrap.
4. Microwave the edamame pods on high for about 2-3 minutes, or until they are heated through.
5. Once cooked, season the edamame pods with salt or other seasonings of your choice, if desired.
6. Serve the edamame pods warm or chilled and enjoy by squeezing the beans out of the pods directly into your mouth.

Seasoning Ideas:
- Sea salt, Soy sauce
- Sesame oil, Chili flakes
- Garlic powder, Lime juice
- Furikake (Japanese seasoning)
- Sriracha sauce

67. Cottage cheese with tomatoes

Ingredients:
- Cottage cheese
- Ripe tomatoes
- Optional: Salt, pepper, olive oil, balsamic vinegar, fresh herbs (such as basil or parsley)

Instructions:
1. Wash the tomatoes thoroughly under running water and pat them dry with a clean towel.

2. Slice the tomatoes into thin rounds or chop them into bite-sized pieces, depending on your preference.

3. Place a generous scoop of cottage cheese onto a serving plate or bowl.

4. Arrange the sliced or chopped tomatoes on top of the cottage cheese.

5. If desired, season the cottage cheese and tomatoes with a pinch of salt and pepper to taste.

6. Drizzle a little olive oil and balsamic vinegar over the cottage cheese and tomatoes for extra flavor, if desired.

7. Garnish the dish with fresh herbs like basil or parsley for a pop of color and added freshness.

8. Serve the cottage cheese with tomatoes immediately and enjoy!

Variations:

- Caprese Style: Layer slices of fresh mozzarella cheese with tomatoes and basil leaves, then drizzle with olive oil and balsamic glaze.
- Spicy Cottage Cheese: Add a sprinkle of red pepper flakes or a dash of hot sauce to the cottage cheese and tomatoes for a spicy kick.
- Herbed Cottage Cheese: Mix chopped fresh herbs like chives, dill, or cilantro into the cottage cheese before topping with tomatoes for added flavor.

Cottage cheese with tomatoes is a versatile dish that can be enjoyed as a light meal, snack, or side dish. It's quick and easy to prepare and provides a good balance of protein, vitamins, and minerals.

68. Trail mix (nuts, seeds, dried fruit)

Basic Trail Mix:
Ingredients:
- 1 cup nuts (such as almonds, cashews, peanuts, walnuts, or pecans)
- 1/2 cup seeds (such as pumpkin seeds, sunflower seeds, or flaxseeds)
- 1/2 cup dried fruit (such as raisins, cranberries, apricots, or cherries)
- Optional: 1/4 cup chocolate chips, coconut flakes, pretzels, or popcorn for added sweetness or crunch

Instructions:
1. In a large mixing bowl, combine the nuts, seeds, dried fruit, and any optional ingredients you'd like to include.

2. Toss the ingredients together until evenly distributed.

3. Transfer the trail mix to an airtight container or portion it out into individual snack bags for easy grab-and-go snacks.

4. Store the trail mix in a cool, dry place until ready to eat.

Variations:

- Sweet and Salty Trail Mix: Combine nuts, seeds, and dried fruit with chocolate chips and pretzels for a delicious sweet and salty flavor combination.

- Tropical Trail Mix: Mix nuts and seeds with dried pineapple, mango, coconut flakes, and banana chips for a taste of the tropics.

- Nut-Free Trail Mix: Use roasted chickpeas, soy nuts, or seeds as the base instead of nuts for a nut-free option that's still packed with protein and fiber.

- Protein-Packed Trail Mix: Add protein-rich ingredients like edamame, roasted chickpeas, or protein-packed cereal to boost the protein content of your trail mix.

- Spicy Trail Mix: Toss nuts and seeds with a sprinkle of chili powder, cayenne pepper, or your favorite spicy seasoning blend for a spicy kick.

Feel free to customize your trail mix with your favorite ingredients to create delicious and satisfying snacks that you'll love to enjoy anytime, anywhere.

69. Cucumber slices with tzatziki

Ingredients:
For the tzatziki:
- 1 cup Greek yogurt
- 1 cucumber, grated and drained
- 2 cloves garlic, minced
- 1 tablespoon fresh lemon juice
- 1 tablespoon extra virgin olive oil
- 1 tablespoon fresh dill, chopped
- Salt and pepper to taste

For serving: 1 cucumber, washed and sliced into rounds or sticks

Instructions:
1. Start by preparing the tzatziki. In a mixing bowl, combine the Greek yogurt, grated and drained cucumber, minced garlic, lemon juice, olive oil, and chopped dill. Mix well to combine.

2. Season the tzatziki with salt and pepper to taste. Adjust the seasoning as needed to suit your preferences.

3. Transfer the tzatziki to a serving bowl and garnish with additional chopped dill, if desired. Cover and refrigerate until ready to serve.

4. Wash the cucumber for serving and slice it into rounds or sticks, depending on your preference.

5. Arrange the cucumber slices or sticks on a serving platter or individual plates. Serve the cucumber slices with the tzatziki dip on the side for dipping. Enjoy your refreshing and delicious snack of cucumber slices with tzatziki!

Variations:
- Minty Tzatziki: Add chopped fresh mint leaves to the tzatziki for a refreshing twist.
- Spicy Tzatziki: Stir in a pinch of cayenne pepper or a dash of hot sauce to the tzatziki for some heat.
- Herbed Tzatziki: Experiment with different herbs such as parsley, cilantro, or basil in addition to or in place of dill.
- Chunky Tzatziki: For a chunkier texture, finely dice the cucumber instead of grating it.

Cucumber slices with tzatziki is a light and refreshing snack that's perfect for serving at parties, picnics, or as a healthy afternoon snack. Enjoy the cool crunch of the cucumber paired with the creamy tanginess of the tzatziki dip!

70. Caprese skewers

Ingredients:
- Fresh mozzarella balls (bocconcini or ciliegine)
- Cherry or grape tomatoes
- Fresh basil leaves
- Balsamic glaze (optional)
- Wooden skewers or toothpicks

Instructions:
1. If you're using wooden skewers, soak them in water for about 30 minutes to prevent them from burning.

2. Wash the cherry or grape tomatoes and pat them dry with a clean towel.

3. Drain the fresh mozzarella balls if they are stored in liquid.

4. Assemble the skewers by threading a tomato, a folded basil leaf, and a mozzarella ball onto each skewer or toothpick. Repeat until all ingredients are used.

5. Arrange the assembled Caprese skewers on a serving platter or dish.

6. If desired, drizzle the skewers with balsamic glaze for extra flavor and visual appeal.

7. Serve the Caprese skewers immediately as a light and refreshing appetizer or snack.

Variations:

- Caprese Salad: If you prefer, you can skip the skewers and arrange the ingredients in layers on a platter or individual plates, drizzling with balsamic glaze before serving.

- Caprese Skewer Salad: Create a salad by mixing additional ingredients such as mixed greens, avocado slices, or cooked quinoa with the Caprese skewers. Toss with a light vinaigrette dressing before serving.

- Caprese Pasta Salad: Combine cooked pasta with halved cherry tomatoes, diced fresh mozzarella, torn basil leaves, and balsamic glaze for a delicious Caprese-inspired pasta salad.

Caprese skewers are a simple yet elegant appetizer that's perfect for entertaining or enjoying as a light snack. They're bursting with fresh flavors and are sure to be a hit with your family and friends!

71. Veggie frittata

Ingredients:
- 8 large eggs
- 1/4 cup milk or heavy cream
- Salt and pepper, to taste
- 2 tablespoons olive oil
- 1 small onion, diced
- 2 cloves garlic, minced
- 2 cups mixed vegetables (such as bell peppers, mushrooms, spinach, zucchini, cherry tomatoes, etc.), chopped
- 1/2 cup shredded cheese (such as cheddar, mozzarella, or feta)
- Fresh herbs (such as parsley, basil, or chives), chopped (optional)

Instructions:

1. Preheat your oven to 375°F (190°C).

2. In a large bowl, whisk together the eggs, milk or cream, salt, and pepper until well combined. Set aside.

3. Heat the olive oil in a 10-inch oven-safe skillet over medium heat. Add the diced onion to the skillet and cook until softened, about 3-4 minutes.

5. Add the minced garlic to the skillet and cook for an additional 1 minute, or until fragrant.

6. Add the mixed vegetables to the skillet and cook until they are tender, about 5-7 minutes.

7. Pour the egg mixture over the vegetables in the skillet, making sure they are evenly distributed.

8. Sprinkle the shredded cheese evenly over the top of the frittata.

9. Transfer the skillet to the preheated oven and bake for 15-20 minutes, or until the frittata is set in the center and lightly golden brown on top.

10. Once cooked, remove the skillet from the oven and let the frittata cool for a few minutes.

11. Garnish the frittata with fresh herbs, if desired, then slice it into wedges and serve.

12. Enjoy your delicious veggie frittata warm or at room temperature as a satisfying breakfast, brunch, or light meal.

Feel free to customize your veggie frittata with your favorite vegetables, cheeses, and herbs to suit your taste preferences. It's a versatile dish that's perfect for using up leftover vegetables and can be enjoyed any time of day!

72. Avocado toast on whole grain

Ingredients:
- 1 ripe avocado
- 2 slices of whole grain bread
- Salt and pepper, to taste
- Optional toppings: sliced tomatoes, red pepper flakes, microgreens, poached or fried egg, crumbled feta cheese, or drizzle of balsamic glaze

Instructions:

1. Start by toasting the whole grain bread slices until they are golden brown and crispy.

2. While the bread is toasting, halve the avocado and remove the pit. Scoop the avocado flesh into a small bowl.

3. Use a fork to mash the avocado until it reaches your desired consistency. You can leave it slightly chunky or mash it until it's smooth.

4. Season the mashed avocado with salt and pepper to taste, and mix well to combine.

5. Once the bread is toasted, spread the mashed avocado evenly onto each slice.

6. If desired, top the avocado toast with additional toppings such as sliced tomatoes, red pepper flakes, microgreens, poached or fried egg, crumbled feta cheese, or a drizzle of balsamic glaze.

7. Serve the avocado toast immediately and enjoy!

Avocado toast on whole grain bread is a versatile dish that can be customized with your favorite toppings to create endless flavor combinations. It's perfect for breakfast, brunch, lunch, or a quick and satisfying snack any time of day.

73. Greek yogurt parfaits

Ingredients:
- Greek yogurt (plain or flavored)
- Granola
- Fresh fruit (such as berries, sliced bananas, diced mango, or kiwi)
- Honey or maple syrup (optional)
- Nuts or seeds (such as almonds, walnuts, pecans, pumpkin seeds, or chia seeds)
- Optional toppings: shredded coconut, dried fruit, cocoa nibs, or a drizzle of nut butter

Instructions:
1. Start by layering the ingredients in a serving glass or bowl. Begin with a spoonful of Greek yogurt at the bottom.

2. Add a layer of granola on top of the Greek yogurt. You can use store-bought granola or make your own at home.

3. Top the granola with a layer of fresh fruit. Choose your favorite fruits or use a combination for added variety and flavor.

4. Drizzle a little honey or maple syrup over the fruit layer for added sweetness, if desired.

5. Add another layer of Greek yogurt on top of the fruit, followed by another layer of granola.

6. Continue layering the ingredients until you reach the top of the serving glass or bowl, finishing with a final layer of Greek yogurt.

7. Garnish the top of the parfait with additional fresh fruit, nuts, seeds, or other toppings of your choice.

8. Serve the Greek yogurt parfait immediately, or cover and refrigerate until ready to eat.

9. Enjoy your delicious and nutritious Greek yogurt parfait as a satisfying breakfast, snack, or dessert option!

Variations:
- Chocolate Lover's Parfait: Add a spoonful of cocoa powder or chocolate chips to the Greek yogurt for a chocolatey twist.
- Tropical Paradise Parfait: Use diced pineapple, mango, and toasted coconut flakes for a taste of the tropics.
- Peanut Butter Banana Parfait: Layer sliced bananas with peanut butter and granola for a deliciously creamy and satisfying parfait.

74. Overnight oats with fruit

Ingredients:
- 1/2 cup rolled oats (old-fashioned oats)
- 1/2 cup Greek yogurt
- 1/2 cup milk (dairy or non-dairy)
- 1 tablespoon chia seeds (optional)
- 1/2 teaspoon vanilla extract (optional)
- Honey or maple syrup, to taste (optional)
- Fresh fruit (such as berries, sliced bananas, diced mango, or chopped apples)
- Additional toppings: nuts, seeds, shredded coconut, or nut butter (optional)

Instructions:

1. In a mason jar or airtight container, combine the rolled oats, Greek yogurt, milk, chia seeds (if using), vanilla extract (if using), and sweetener (if using). Stir well to combine all ingredients.

2. Add a layer of fresh fruit on top of the oat mixture. Choose your favorite fruits or use a combination for added variety and flavor.

3. Seal the jar or container tightly with a lid and shake gently to mix the ingredients together.

4. Place the overnight oats in the refrigerator and let them chill for at least 4 hours or overnight to allow the oats to soften and absorb the liquid.

5. In the morning, give the overnight oats a stir to evenly distribute the fruit and toppings.

6. If desired, top the overnight oats with additional fresh fruit, nuts, seeds, shredded coconut, or nut butter before serving.

7. Enjoy your delicious and nutritious overnight oats with fruit straight from the refrigerator or let them sit at room temperature for a few minutes to take off the chill.

Variations:
- Chocolate Banana Overnight Oats: Add a tablespoon of cocoa powder and sliced bananas to the overnight oats for a chocolatey treat.
- Apple Cinnamon Overnight Oats: Stir in diced apples and a sprinkle of cinnamon to the overnight oats for a cozy and comforting flavor.
- Berry Blast Overnight Oats: Use a mix of your favorite berries (such as strawberries, blueberries, raspberries, and blackberries) for a burst of color and antioxidants.
- Tropical Overnight Oats: Use diced pineapple, mango, and toasted coconut flakes for a taste of the tropics.

75. Tofu scramble with veggies

Ingredients:
- 1 block of firm tofu
- 1 tablespoon olive oil
- 1 small onion, diced
- 2 cloves garlic, minced
- 1 bell pepper, diced
- 1 cup of mushrooms, sliced
- 1 cup of spinach or kale, chopped
- 2 tablespoons nutritional yeast (optional, for a cheesy flavor)
- 1 teaspoon turmeric powder (for color and flavor)
- Salt and pepper to taste
- Optional toppings: avocado slices, chopped tomatoes, salsa, hot sauce

Instructions:
1. Start by pressing the tofu to remove excess moisture. Wrap the block of tofu in paper towels and place it between two plates. Place a heavy object, like a can or a skillet, on top of the plate to press down on the tofu. Let it sit for about 15-20 minutes.

2. While the tofu is pressing, prepare your veggies. Dice the onion, mince the garlic, chop the bell pepper, slice the mushrooms, and chop the spinach or kale.

3. Once the tofu is pressed, crumble it into a bowl using your hands or a fork to achieve a scrambled egg-like texture.

4. Heat olive oil in a large skillet over medium heat. Add the diced onion and minced garlic, and sauté for 2-3 minutes until fragrant.

5. Add the diced bell pepper and sliced mushrooms to the skillet. Cook for another 5-7 minutes until the vegetables are tender.

6. Add the crumbled tofu to the skillet, along with the nutritional yeast (if using), turmeric powder, salt, and pepper. Stir well to combine and evenly distribute the seasonings.

7. Cook the tofu scramble for an additional 5-7 minutes, stirring occasionally, until the tofu is heated through and slightly golden.

8. Add the chopped spinach or kale to the skillet and cook for another 2-3 minutes until wilted.

9. Taste and adjust seasoning if necessary. Serve hot, garnished with your favorite toppings such as avocado slices, chopped tomatoes, salsa, or hot sauce.

76. Whole grain waffles with nut butter

Ingredients:
- 1 cup whole wheat flour
- 1/2 cup rolled oats
- 1 tablespoon baking powder
- 1 tablespoon sugar or maple syrup (optional)
- 1/2 teaspoon salt
- 1 cup milk (dairy or plant-based)
- 1/4 cup melted butter or oil
- 1 teaspoon vanilla extract
- Nut butter of your choice (such as peanut butter, almond butter, or cashew butter)
- Optional toppings: sliced bananas, berries, chopped nuts, honey, or maple syrup

Instructions:
1. In a large mixing bowl, combine the whole wheat flour, rolled oats, baking powder, sugar (if using), and salt. Stir until well mixed.

2. In a separate bowl, whisk together the milk, melted butter or oil, and vanilla extract.

3. Pour the wet ingredients into the dry ingredients and stir until just combined. Be careful not to overmix; a few lumps are okay.

4. Preheat your waffle iron according to the manufacturer's instructions.

5. Once the waffle iron is hot, lightly grease it with non-stick cooking spray or brush it with a little melted butter or oil.

6. Pour enough batter onto the waffle iron to cover the surface (the amount will depend on the size of your waffle iron). Close the lid and cook according to the manufacturer's instructions, usually for 3-5 minutes, or until the waffles are golden brown and crispy.

7. Carefully remove the cooked waffles from the waffle iron and repeat with the remaining batter.

8. Once all the waffles are cooked, spread a generous amount of nut butter on each waffle.

9. Serve the whole grain waffles with nut butter hot, garnished with your favorite toppings such as sliced bananas, berries, chopped nuts, honey, or maple syrup.

Enjoy your delicious and wholesome whole grain waffles with nut butter!

77. Smoked salmon on whole wheat toast

Ingredients:
- Slices of whole wheat bread
- Smoked salmon slices
- Cream cheese or Greek yogurt (optional)
- Thinly sliced red onion (optional)
- Capers (optional)
- Fresh dill or chives, chopped (optional)
- Lemon wedges (optional)
- Salt and pepper to taste

Instructions:
1. Toast the slices of whole wheat bread until they are golden brown and crispy.

2. If desired, spread a thin layer of cream cheese or Greek yogurt onto the toasted bread slices. This adds a creamy texture and enhances the flavor of the smoked salmon.

3. Arrange slices of smoked salmon on top of the toast. You can layer them neatly or fold them into attractive shapes.

4. If using, add thinly sliced red onion on top of the smoked salmon. Red onion adds a sharp and slightly sweet flavor that complements the richness of the salmon.

5. Sprinkle capers over the smoked salmon. Capers provide a burst of briny flavor that pairs well with the smokiness of the salmon.

6. Garnish with chopped fresh dill or chives for added freshness and a pop of color.

7. Squeeze lemon wedges over the smoked salmon to add a touch of brightness and acidity. Lemon juice enhances the flavors of the dish and balances the richness of the salmon.

8. Season with salt and pepper to taste.

9. Serve the smoked salmon on whole wheat toast immediately, either as an elegant breakfast or brunch option.

Enjoy your delicious smoked salmon on whole wheat toast!

78. Chia pudding with berries

Ingredients:
- 1/4 cup chia seeds
- 1 cup milk of your choice (dairy milk, almond milk, coconut milk, etc.)
- 1-2 tablespoons sweetener of your choice (such as honey, maple syrup, agave nectar, or sugar), optional
- 1/2 teaspoon vanilla extract
- Fresh berries (such as strawberries, blueberries, raspberries, or blackberries), washed and sliced
- Optional toppings: sliced almonds, shredded coconut, granola, or additional berries

Instructions:

1. In a mixing bowl or jar, combine the chia seeds, milk, sweetener (if using), and vanilla extract. Stir well to combine.

2. Let the mixture sit for a few minutes, then stir again to prevent clumping. Cover the bowl or jar and refrigerate for at least 2 hours or overnight. The chia seeds will absorb the liquid and thicken to form a pudding-like consistency.

3. After the chia pudding has chilled and thickened, give it a good stir to break up any clumps.

4. Divide the chia pudding into serving bowls or glasses.

5. Top the chia pudding with fresh berries of your choice. You can use a single type of berry or a combination for a colorful and flavorful topping.

6. Add any optional toppings you like, such as sliced almonds, shredded coconut, granola, or additional berries.

7. Serve the chia pudding with berries immediately, or cover and refrigerate until ready to serve.

8. Enjoy your delicious and nutritious chia pudding with berries as a refreshing dessert or breakfast option!

Feel free to adjust the sweetness level according to your taste preferences by adding more or less sweetener. You can also customize the toppings based on your favorite flavors and textures.

79. Egg white veggie omelet

Ingredients:
- 4 egg whites
- 1/4 cup diced bell peppers (any color)
- 1/4 cup diced tomatoes
- 1/4 cup diced onions
- 1/4 cup chopped spinach or kale
- Salt and pepper to taste
- Cooking spray or olive oil

Optional additions:
- Sliced mushrooms
- Diced zucchini
- Chopped broccoli
- Crumbled feta cheese
- Fresh herbs like parsley or chives

Instructions:

1. In a small bowl, whisk the egg whites until frothy. You can also season them with a pinch of salt and pepper if desired.

2. Heat a non-stick skillet over medium heat and lightly coat it with cooking spray or olive oil.

3. Add the diced bell peppers, tomatoes, onions, and any other vegetables you're using to the skillet. Sauté them for a few minutes until they are tender but still crisp.

4. Add the chopped spinach or kale to the skillet and cook for another minute until wilted. Season the veggies with a pinch of salt and pepper.

5. Pour the whisked egg whites evenly over the cooked vegetables in the skillet.

6. Allow the eggs to cook undisturbed for a minute or two until the edges start to set.

7. Gently lift the edges of the omelet with a spatula and tilt the skillet to let the uncooked egg flow to the edges.

8. Once the omelet is mostly set but still slightly runny on top, carefully fold it in half using the spatula.

9. Cook for another minute or until the egg whites are fully set and the omelet is lightly golden on both sides.

10. Slide the omelet onto a plate and garnish with any additional toppings you like, such as fresh herbs or crumbled feta cheese. Serve the egg white veggie omelet hot and enjoy a nutritious and delicious breakfast!

Feel free to customize the omelet with your favorite vegetables and toppings to suit your taste preferences. It's a versatile dish that can be enjoyed any time of day!

80. Steel cut oatmeal with fruit

Ingredients:
- 1 cup steel-cut oats
- 3 cups water
- Pinch of salt
- Fresh fruit of your choice (such as berries, sliced bananas, chopped apples, or diced peaches)
- Optional toppings: chopped nuts, seeds, honey, maple syrup, cinnamon, or yogurt

Instructions:

1. In a medium-sized saucepan, bring 3 cups of water to a boil.

2. Add a pinch of salt to the boiling water.

3. Stir in the steel-cut oats and reduce the heat to low.

4. Simmer the oats uncovered, stirring occasionally, for about 20-30 minutes or until they reach your desired consistency. Steel-cut oats have a chewier texture compared to rolled oats, so they may take longer to cook.

5. While the oats are cooking, prepare your fruit toppings. Wash and chop your chosen fruits into bite-sized pieces.

6. Once the oats are cooked to your liking, remove the saucepan from the heat.

7. Serve the steel-cut oatmeal hot in bowls, topped with your favorite fresh fruit.

8. Add any additional toppings you desire, such as chopped nuts, seeds, honey, maple syrup, cinnamon, or a dollop of yogurt.

9. Give the oatmeal a gentle stir to incorporate the toppings.

10. Enjoy your delicious and nutritious steel-cut oatmeal with fruit for a satisfying breakfast that will keep you fueled throughout the morning!

Feel free to customize your oatmeal with different fruit combinations and toppings to suit your taste preferences. You can also make a larger batch of steel-cut oats and store the leftovers in the refrigerator for easy reheating on busy mornings.

81. Dark chocolate avocado mousse

Ingredients:
- 2 ripe avocados
- 1/4 cup cocoa powder (unsweetened)
- 1/4 cup maple syrup or honey (adjust to taste)
- 1 teaspoon vanilla extract
- Pinch of salt
- Optional toppings: shaved dark chocolate, sliced strawberries, raspberries, or whipped coconut cream

Instructions:

1. Cut the avocados in half, remove the pits, and scoop the flesh into a blender or food processor.

2. Add the cocoa powder, maple syrup or honey, vanilla extract, and a pinch of salt to the blender.

3. Blend the ingredients until smooth and creamy, scraping down the sides of the blender or food processor as needed to ensure everything is well incorporated. Taste the mousse and adjust the sweetness if necessary by adding more maple syrup or honey.

4. Once the mousse is smooth and creamy, transfer it to serving dishes or small bowls.

5. Refrigerate the mousse for at least 30 minutes to chill and firm up slightly.

6. Before serving, garnish the dark chocolate avocado mousse with your choice of toppings, such as shaved dark chocolate, sliced strawberries, raspberries, or a dollop of whipped coconut cream.

7. Serve the mousse chilled and enjoy its rich, creamy texture and indulgent chocolate flavor!

This dark chocolate avocado mousse is a great alternative to traditional mousse recipes that are loaded with sugar and heavy cream. It's naturally sweetened with maple syrup or honey and gets its creamy texture from the avocado. Plus, it's packed with healthy fats and antioxidants, making it a guilt-free dessert option.

82. Baked apples with cinnamon

Ingredients:
- 4 medium-sized apples (such as Granny Smith, Honeycrisp, or Fuji)
- 2 tablespoons butter or coconut oil, melted
- 2 tablespoons brown sugar or coconut sugar (optional, adjust to taste)
- 1 teaspoon ground cinnamon
- Pinch of nutmeg (optional)
- Pinch of salt
- Optional toppings: vanilla ice cream, whipped cream, chopped nuts, or caramel sauce

Instructions:
1. Preheat your oven to 375°F (190°C).

2. Wash the apples and pat them dry. Using an apple corer or a sharp knife, remove the cores from the apples, leaving the bottoms intact to create a well for the filling.

3. In a small bowl, mix together the melted butter or coconut oil, brown sugar or coconut sugar (if using), ground cinnamon, nutmeg (if using), and a pinch of salt.

4. Place the cored apples in a baking dish or oven-safe skillet.

5. Spoon the cinnamon mixture evenly into the wells of the apples, filling them to the top.

6. If desired, sprinkle a little extra cinnamon on top of each apple for added flavor.

7. Cover the baking dish or skillet with foil and bake in the preheated oven for 25-30 minutes, or until the apples are tender but not mushy. The baking time may vary depending on the size and variety of apples used.

8. Once the apples are baked, remove them from the oven and let them cool slightly before serving.

9. Serve the baked apples warm, either on their own or with your choice of toppings such as vanilla ice cream, whipped cream, chopped nuts, or caramel sauce.

10. Enjoy the cozy and comforting flavors of baked apples with cinnamon as a delightful dessert or sweet treat!

These baked apples with cinnamon are not only delicious but also fragrant, filling your kitchen with the inviting aroma of warm spices. They're perfect for a cozy dessert on a chilly evening or as a sweet ending to any meal.

83. Chia seed pudding

Ingredients:
- 1/4 cup chia seeds
- 1 cup milk of your choice (dairy milk, almond milk, coconut milk, etc.)
- 1-2 tablespoons sweetener of your choice (such as honey, maple syrup, agave nectar, or sugar), optional
- 1/2 teaspoon vanilla extract
- Optional toppings: fresh fruit, nuts, seeds, granola, shredded coconut, or chocolate chips

Instructions:

1. In a mixing bowl or jar, combine the chia seeds, milk, sweetener (if using), and vanilla extract. Stir well to combine.

2. Let the mixture sit for a few minutes, then stir again to prevent clumping. Cover the bowl or jar and refrigerate for at least 2 hours or overnight. The chia seeds will absorb the liquid and thicken to form a pudding-like consistency.

3. After the chia seed pudding has chilled and thickened, give it a good stir to break up any clumps.

4. Divide the chia seed pudding into serving bowls or glasses.

5. Top the chia seed pudding with your favorite toppings, such as fresh fruit, nuts, seeds, granola, shredded coconut, or chocolate chips.

6. Serve the chia seed pudding immediately, or cover and refrigerate until ready to serve.

7. Enjoy your delicious and nutritious chia seed pudding as a satisfying breakfast, snack, or dessert!

Feel free to customize your chia seed pudding with different types of milk, sweeteners, and toppings to suit your taste preferences. Experiment with various flavor combinations to create your own unique variations of this healthy and delicious dish!

84. Coconut chia parfait

Ingredients:
- 1/4 cup chia seeds
- 1 cup coconut milk (canned or homemade)
- 1-2 tablespoons maple syrup or honey, to taste
- 1/2 teaspoon vanilla extract
- 1/2 cup coconut yogurt or Greek yogurt
- 1/2 cup fresh mixed berries (such as strawberries, blueberries, and raspberries)
- 1/4 cup shredded coconut, toasted (optional)
- Mint leaves for garnish (optional)

Instructions:
1. In a mixing bowl or jar, combine the chia seeds, coconut milk, maple syrup or honey, and vanilla extract. Stir well to combine.

2. Let the mixture sit for a few minutes, then stir again to prevent clumping. Cover the bowl or jar and refrigerate for at least 2 hours or overnight, allowing the chia seeds to absorb the liquid and thicken to a pudding-like consistency.

3. Once the coconut chia pudding has chilled and thickened, give it a good stir to break up any clumps.

4. To assemble the coconut chia parfait, layer the coconut chia pudding and coconut yogurt in serving glasses or jars, alternating between the two layers.

5. Top the parfait with fresh mixed berries and toasted shredded coconut, if desired.

6. Garnish with mint leaves for a fresh touch, if desired.

7. Serve the coconut chia parfait immediately, or cover and refrigerate until ready to serve.

8. Enjoy your delicious and nutritious coconut chia parfait as a refreshing breakfast, snack, or dessert!

This coconut chia parfait is not only tasty but also packed with healthy fats, fiber, and antioxidants. It's a versatile dish that can be customized with your favorite toppings and enjoyed any time of day.

85. Grilled pineapple with cinnamon

Ingredients:
- 1 pineapple, peeled, cored, and cut into slices or wedges
- 1-2 tablespoons honey or maple syrup (optional)
- 1 teaspoon ground cinnamon
- Pinch of salt
- Optional toppings: vanilla ice cream, whipped cream, chopped nuts, or fresh mint leaves

Instructions:
1. Preheat your grill to medium-high heat.

2. In a small bowl, mix together the honey or maple syrup (if using), ground cinnamon, and a pinch of salt.

3. Brush the pineapple slices or wedges with the cinnamon mixture, coating them evenly on both sides.

4. Place the pineapple slices directly on the preheated grill.

5. Grill the pineapple for 2-3 minutes on each side, or until grill marks form and the pineapple is caramelized and slightly softened.

6. Remove the grilled pineapple from the grill and transfer it to a serving platter.

7. If desired, drizzle any remaining cinnamon mixture over the grilled pineapple for extra flavor.

8. Serve the grilled pineapple hot, either on its own or with your choice of toppings such as vanilla ice cream, whipped cream, chopped nuts, or fresh mint leaves.

9. Enjoy the delicious combination of grilled pineapple with cinnamon as a tasty and refreshing dessert!

Grilled pineapple with cinnamon is a simple yet elegant dessert that's perfect for summer gatherings, barbecues, or anytime you're craving something sweet and tropical. The caramelization from grilling enhances the pineapple's natural sweetness, while the cinnamon adds warmth and depth of flavor.

86. Strawberry chia jam bars

Ingredients:
For the strawberry chia jam:
- 2 cups fresh strawberries, hulled and chopped
- 2 tablespoons maple syrup or honey
- 2 tablespoons chia seeds
- 1 teaspoon vanilla extract

For the oatmeal crust and topping:
- 1 1/2 cups rolled oats
- 1/2 cup almond flour or all-purpose flour
- 1/4 cup coconut oil, melted
- 1/4 cup maple syrup or honey
- 1/2 teaspoon vanilla extract
- Pinch of salt

Instructions:

1. Preheat your oven to 350°F (175°C). Grease or line an 8x8 inch baking pan with parchment paper, leaving some overhang on the sides for easy removal.

2. Start by making the strawberry chia jam. In a saucepan, combine the chopped strawberries and maple syrup or honey. Cook over medium heat, stirring occasionally, until the strawberries break down and become soft, about 5-7 minutes.

3. Once the strawberries are soft, mash them with a fork or potato masher to desired consistency. Stir in the chia seeds and vanilla extract, then remove the saucepan from the heat. Let the jam cool and thicken for about 10-15 minutes.

4. In a mixing bowl, combine the rolled oats, almond flour or all-purpose flour, melted coconut oil, maple syrup or honey, vanilla extract, and a pinch of salt. Mix until well combined and the mixture resembles coarse crumbs.

5. Press half of the oatmeal mixture firmly into the bottom of the prepared baking pan, forming an even layer.

6. Spread the cooled strawberry chia jam evenly over the oatmeal crust. Sprinkle the remaining oatmeal mixture evenly over the strawberry chia jam, covering it completely.

7. Bake in the preheated oven for 25-30 minutes, or until the top is golden brown and the edges are slightly crisp.

8. Remove the pan from the oven and let the bars cool completely in the pan on a wire rack.

9. Once cooled, use the parchment paper overhang to lift the bars out of the pan. Place them on a cutting board and slice into bars or squares.

10. Serve the strawberry chia jam bars as a delicious and wholesome snack or dessert. Enjoy your homemade strawberry chia jam bars! Store any leftovers in an airtight container in the refrigerator for up to one week.

87. Dark chocolate dipped fruits

Ingredients:
- Assorted fruits of your choice (such as strawberries, bananas, pineapple chunks, orange slices, or dried apricots)
- Dark chocolate chips or chopped dark chocolate
- Optional toppings: chopped nuts, shredded coconut, or sea salt flakes

Instructions:
1. Wash and dry the fruits thoroughly. If using strawberries, make sure to remove the stems.

2. Line a baking sheet or tray with parchment paper.

3. In a microwave-safe bowl, melt the dark chocolate chips or chopped dark chocolate in the microwave in 30-second intervals, stirring well between each interval, until smooth and fully melted. Alternatively, you can melt the chocolate using a double boiler on the stove.

4. Once the chocolate is melted and smooth, hold each piece of fruit by its stem or with a toothpick and dip it into the melted chocolate, coating it halfway or fully, depending on your preference.

5. Allow any excess chocolate to drip off, then place the chocolate-dipped fruit onto the prepared baking sheet or tray.

6. If desired, sprinkle the chocolate-dipped fruits with chopped nuts, shredded coconut, or a pinch of sea salt flakes while the chocolate is still wet.

7. Repeat the dipping process with the remaining fruits until all are coated in chocolate.

8. Place the baking sheet or tray in the refrigerator for about 15-20 minutes, or until the chocolate has hardened.

9. Once the chocolate has set, remove the chocolate-dipped fruits from the refrigerator. Serve the dark chocolate dipped fruits immediately as a delicious snack or dessert.

10. Enjoy your homemade dark chocolate dipped fruits! Store any leftovers in an airtight container in the refrigerator for up to a few days.

These dark chocolate dipped fruits are not only delicious but also make for an elegant and impressive treat for parties, gatherings, or special occasions. They're perfect for satisfying your sweet tooth while also enjoying the natural goodness of fruits and the antioxidant benefits of dark chocolate.

88. Banana nice cream

Ingredients:
- 2 ripe bananas, peeled and sliced
- Optional add-ins: cocoa powder, peanut butter, vanilla extract, honey, or any other flavorings you like

Instructions:

1. Place the sliced bananas in a microwave-safe bowl.

2. Microwave the bananas on high for 1-2 minutes, or until they are soft and slightly mushy.

3. Carefully transfer the microwaved bananas to a blender or food processor.

4. Add any desired add-ins, such as cocoa powder, peanut butter, vanilla extract, or honey, to the blender or food processor.

5. Blend the bananas and add-ins until smooth and creamy, scraping down the sides of the blender or food processor as needed.

6. Once the mixture is smooth and creamy, transfer it to a container and freeze for at least 2 hours, or until firm.

7. Once the banana nice cream is frozen, scoop it into bowls and serve immediately.

8. Enjoy your delicious and healthy banana nice cream!

This microwave method is a quick and convenient way to make banana nice cream, but keep in mind that the texture may not be as smooth as when using a traditional blender or food processor. Feel free to experiment with different add-ins and toppings to customize your banana nice cream to your liking!

89. Baked stuffed apples

Ingredients:
- 4 large apples
 (such as Granny Smith or Honeycrisp)
- 1/4 cup rolled oats
- 1/4 cup chopped nuts
(such as walnuts or pecans)
- 2 tablespoons brown sugar or maple syrup
- 1 teaspoon ground cinnamon
- Pinch of nutmeg
- 2 tablespoons butter or coconut oil, melted
- Optional toppings: vanilla ice cream, whipped cream, caramel sauce, or a drizzle of honey

Instructions:

1. Preheat your oven to 375°F (190°C). Grease a baking dish large enough to hold the apples.

2. Wash the apples and pat them dry. Using an apple corer or a sharp knife, remove the cores from the apples, leaving the bottoms intact to create a well for the filling. Place the cored apples in the prepared baking dish.

3. In a mixing bowl, combine the rolled oats, chopped nuts, brown sugar or maple syrup, ground cinnamon, and pinch of nutmeg. Stir until well combined.

4. Pour the melted butter or coconut oil over the oat mixture and stir until evenly coated.

5. Spoon the oat mixture into the wells of the cored apples, dividing it evenly among them and pressing it down gently.

6. Cover the baking dish with foil and bake in the preheated oven for 25-30 minutes, or until the apples are tender when pierced with a fork and the filling is golden brown and bubbly.

7. Remove the foil from the baking dish and bake for an additional 5-10 minutes, or until the tops of the apples are lightly browned.

8. Once baked, remove the stuffed apples from the oven and let them cool for a few minutes before serving.

9. Serve the baked stuffed apples warm, optionally topped with vanilla ice cream, whipped cream, caramel sauce, or a drizzle of honey. Enjoy your delicious and comforting baked stuffed apples as a cozy dessert!

These baked stuffed apples are simple to make yet incredibly satisfying, with a warm and spiced filling that pairs perfectly with the tender, sweet apples. They're sure to become a favorite dessert for fall and beyond!

90. Coconut yogurt cups with berries

Ingredients:
- 2 cups coconut yogurt (store-bought or homemade)
- 1 cup mixed berries (such as strawberries, blueberries, raspberries, and blackberries)
- Optional toppings: shredded coconut, chopped nuts, honey, or maple syrup

Instructions:
1. Divide the coconut yogurt evenly among serving cups or bowls.

2. Wash the mixed berries and pat them dry. If using strawberries, remove the stems and slice them into bite-sized pieces.

3. Top each coconut yogurt cup with a generous portion of mixed berries.

4. If desired, sprinkle shredded coconut and chopped nuts over the berries for added texture and flavor.

5. Drizzle honey or maple syrup over the yogurt cups for a touch of sweetness, if desired.

6. Serve the coconut yogurt cups with berries immediately as a refreshing snack or dessert.

7. Enjoy your delicious and nutritious coconut yogurt cups with berries!

These coconut yogurt cups with berries are not only tasty but also packed with antioxidants, vitamins, and probiotics. They make for a satisfying and wholesome treat that's perfect for any time of day. Feel free to customize the toppings based on your preferences or what's available seasonally.

91. Extra virgin olive oil

Extra virgin olive oil is a type of oil that's made from the pressing of olives. It's widely regarded as one of the healthiest oils due to its high content of monounsaturated fats, antioxidants, and other beneficial compounds. Here are some key points about extra virgin olive oil:

1. Health Benefits: Extra virgin olive oil is rich in monounsaturated fats, particularly oleic acid, which is associated with numerous health benefits, including reduced risk of heart disease and improved cholesterol levels. It also contains antioxidants, such as vitamin E and polyphenols, which have anti-inflammatory and protective properties.

2. Types of Olive Oil: Olive oil is available in several grades, with extra virgin olive oil being the highest quality and most flavorful. It is obtained from the first pressing of olives and undergoes minimal processing, preserving its natural taste and nutritional value. Other types of olive oil include virgin olive oil, which is also obtained from the first pressing but has slightly higher acidity levels, and refined olive oil, which is processed to remove impurities and has a milder flavor.

3. Flavor Profile: Extra virgin olive oil has a distinct flavor profile that can range from fruity and grassy to peppery and bitter, depending on factors such as the variety of olives used, the region of production, and the harvesting and processing methods. It's commonly used as a finishing oil to drizzle over salads, vegetables, bread, and grilled meats, as well as in dressings, marinades, and sauces.

4. Cooking Uses: While extra virgin olive oil is prized for its flavor and nutritional benefits, it has a lower smoke point compared to some other cooking oils, such as canola or avocado oil. This means it's best suited for low to medium-heat cooking methods, such as sautéing, roasting, and baking. It's not recommended for high-heat cooking techniques like deep-frying, as exposure to high temperatures can degrade its flavor and nutritional properties.

5. Storage and Shelf Life: To maintain the quality of extra virgin olive oil, it's important to store it properly in a cool, dark place away from heat and light, as exposure to air, light, and heat can cause it to oxidize and spoil more quickly. When stored correctly, extra virgin olive oil can have a shelf life of up to two years or more.

Overall, extra virgin olive oil is a versatile and flavorful oil that's not only delicious but also offers a range of health benefits when consumed as part of a balanced diet.

92. Avocado oil

1. Avocado Oil Vinaigrette:
  - 1/4 cup avocado oil
  - 2 tbsp vinegar
  - 1 tsp Dijon mustard
  - 1 clove minced garlic
  - Salt and pepper to taste

Instructions: Whisk all ingredients together. Store in fridge for up to a week.

2. Avocado Oil Roasted Vegetables:
  - Assorted vegetables
  - 2-3 tbsp avocado oil
  - Salt, pepper, and optional seasonings

Instructions: Toss vegetables with oil and seasonings. Roast at 400°F for 20-25 mins.

3. Avocado Oil Garlic Herb Salmon:
  - 4 salmon fillets
  - 2 tbsp avocado oil
  - 2 cloves minced garlic
  - 1 tsp dried herbs
  - Salt and pepper to taste

Instructions: Brush salmon with oil mixture. Bake at 400°F for 12-15 mins.

93. Balsamic vinaigrette

Ingredients:
- 1/4 cup balsamic vinegar
- 1/2 cup extra virgin olive oil
- 1 tablespoon Dijon mustard
- 1 clove garlic, minced (optional)
- 1 teaspoon honey or maple syrup (optional)
- Salt and pepper to taste

Instructions:
1. In a small bowl or jar, whisk together the balsamic vinegar, Dijon mustard, minced garlic (if using), honey or maple syrup (if using), salt, and pepper until well combined.

2. Gradually pour in the extra virgin olive oil while whisking continuously, until the vinaigrette is emulsified and thickened.

3. Taste and adjust the seasoning, adding more salt, pepper, or sweetener if desired.

4. Use the balsamic vinaigrette immediately, or store it in an airtight container in the refrigerator for up to one week. Shake well before serving.

Enjoy your homemade balsamic vinaigrette drizzled over salads, roasted vegetables, grilled meats, or as a marinade for chicken or tofu!

94. Tahini dressing

Ingredients:
- 1/4 cup tahini
- 2 tablespoons lemon juice
- 2 tablespoons water
- 1 clove garlic, minced (optional)
- 1 teaspoon honey or maple syrup (optional)
- Salt and pepper to taste

Instructions:
1. In a small bowl, whisk together the tahini, lemon juice, water, minced garlic (if using), honey or maple syrup (if using), salt, and pepper until smooth and creamy.

2. If the dressing is too thick, add more water, a tablespoon at a time, until you reach your desired consistency.

3. Taste and adjust the seasoning, adding more salt, pepper, lemon juice, or sweetener if desired.

4. Use the tahini dressing immediately, or store it in an airtight container in the refrigerator for up to one week. Stir well before serving.

Enjoy your homemade tahini dressing drizzled over salads, grain bowls, roasted vegetables, falafel, or as a dip for raw veggies!

95. Walnut oil vinaigrette

Ingredients:
- 1/4 cup walnut oil
- 2 tablespoons white wine vinegar or apple cider vinegar
- 1 teaspoon Dijon mustard
- 1 teaspoon honey or maple syrup (optional)
- Salt and pepper to taste

Instructions:

1. In a small bowl or jar, whisk together the walnut oil, white wine vinegar or apple cider vinegar, Dijon mustard, honey or maple syrup (if using), salt, and pepper until well combined.

2. Taste and adjust the seasoning, adding more salt, pepper, or sweetener if desired.

3. Use the walnut oil vinaigrette immediately, or store it in an airtight container in the refrigerator for up to one week. Shake well before serving.

Enjoy your homemade walnut oil vinaigrette drizzled over salads, roasted vegetables, grilled meats, or as a marinade for chicken or tofu!

96. Chimichurri sauce

Chimichurri sauce is a vibrant and flavorful condiment that originates from Argentina. It's traditionally served with grilled meats but can also be used as a marinade or topping for various dishes. Here's a classic recipe:

Ingredients:
- 1 cup fresh parsley, finely chopped
- 1/4 cup fresh cilantro, finely chopped
- 3 cloves garlic, minced
- 1 shallot, finely chopped (optional)
- 1/4 cup red wine vinegar or white wine vinegar
- 1/2 cup extra virgin olive oil
- 1 tablespoon dried oregano
- 1 teaspoon red pepper flakes (adjust to taste)
- Salt and pepper to taste
- 1 tablespoon lemon juice (optional)

Instructions:
1. In a mixing bowl, combine the chopped parsley, chopped cilantro, minced garlic, and chopped shallot (if using).

2. Add the red wine vinegar or white wine vinegar, extra virgin olive oil, dried oregano, red pepper flakes, salt, and pepper to the bowl.

3. Stir the ingredients together until well combined.

4. Taste the chimichurri sauce and adjust the seasoning as needed, adding more salt, pepper, or red pepper flakes to taste. If you prefer a tangier sauce, you can also add a tablespoon of lemon juice.

5. Let the chimichurri sauce sit at room temperature for at least 15-30 minutes to allow the flavors to meld together before serving.

6. Serve the chimichurri sauce alongside grilled meats, such as steak, chicken, or pork, or use it as a marinade or topping for other dishes.

Enjoy the fresh and herbaceous flavors of chimichurri sauce with your favorite grilled meats or other dishes! Unused chimichurri sauce can be stored in an airtight container in the refrigerator for up to one week.

97. Pesto with walnuts or hemp seeds

Ingredients:
- 2 cups fresh basil leaves, packed
- 1/2 cup walnuts or hemp seeds (shelled)
- 2 cloves garlic, peeled
- 1/2 cup grated Parmesan cheese (optional, omit for vegan version)
- 1/2 cup extra virgin olive oil
- Salt and pepper to taste
- Squeeze of lemon juice (optional)

Instructions:
1. In a food processor, combine the fresh basil leaves, walnuts or hemp seeds, and peeled garlic cloves.

2. Pulse until the ingredients are finely chopped and well combined.

3. Add the grated Parmesan cheese (if using) to the food processor and pulse a few more times to incorporate.

4. With the food processor running, slowly drizzle in the extra virgin olive oil until the pesto reaches your desired consistency. You may need to stop and scrape down the sides of the food processor with a spatula as needed.

5. Season the pesto with salt and pepper to taste. If you'd like a bit of brightness, you can also add a squeeze of lemon juice at this stage.

6. Continue to blend until the pesto is smooth and well combined.

7. Taste the pesto and adjust the seasoning, adding more salt, pepper, or lemon juice if needed.

8. Transfer the pesto to a jar or container with a tight-fitting lid. If not using immediately, store the pesto in the refrigerator for up to one week.

Enjoy your homemade pesto with walnuts or hemp seeds tossed with pasta, spread on sandwiches, used as a pizza topping, or incorporated into various recipes for a burst of fresh flavor!

98. Greek yogurt ranch dressing

Ingredients:
- 1 cup plain Greek yogurt
- 1/4 cup mayonnaise
- 2 tablespoons fresh lemon juice
- 2 cloves garlic, minced
- 2 tablespoons chopped fresh parsley
- 1 tablespoon chopped fresh dill (or 1 teaspoon dried dill)
- 1 teaspoon onion powder
- 1 teaspoon dried chives
- 1/2 teaspoon paprika
- Salt and pepper to taste

Instructions:

1. In a mixing bowl, combine the plain Greek yogurt, mayonnaise, and fresh lemon juice. Stir until smooth and well combined.

2. Add the minced garlic, chopped fresh parsley, chopped fresh dill (or dried dill), onion powder, dried chives, paprika, salt, and pepper to the bowl.

3. Stir the ingredients together until the herbs and spices are evenly distributed throughout the dressing.

4. Taste the Greek yogurt ranch dressing and adjust the seasoning as needed, adding more salt, pepper, or lemon juice if desired.

5. If the dressing is too thick, you can thin it out with a little water until you reach your desired consistency.

6. Transfer the Greek yogurt ranch dressing to a jar or container with a tight-fitting lid. Store it in the refrigerator for up to one week.

Enjoy your homemade Greek yogurt ranch dressing drizzled over salads, used as a dip for veggies, or as a flavorful topping for baked potatoes or grilled meats!

99. Mango salsa

Ingredients:
- 2 ripe mangos, diced
- 1/2 red onion, finely chopped
- 1 red bell pepper, diced
- 1 jalapeño pepper, seeded and minced
- 1/4 cup fresh cilantro, chopped
- Juice of 1 lime
- Salt and pepper to taste

Instructions:

1. In a mixing bowl, combine the diced mango, finely chopped red onion, diced red bell pepper, minced jalapeño pepper, and chopped fresh cilantro.

2. Squeeze the juice of one lime over the mango salsa mixture.

3. Season the salsa with salt and pepper to taste.

4. Gently toss all the ingredients together until well combined.

5. Taste the mango salsa and adjust the seasoning as needed, adding more salt, pepper, or lime juice if desired.

6. Serve the mango salsa immediately, or cover and refrigerate it for at least 30 minutes to allow the flavors to meld together before serving.

Enjoy your homemade mango salsa as a refreshing dip with tortilla chips, or as a topping for grilled fish, chicken, tacos, or salads! Adjust the spiciness level by adding more or less jalapeño pepper, depending on your preference.

100. Tzatziki sauce

Ingredients:
- 1 cucumber, grated
- 1 1/2 cups plain Greek yogurt
- 2 cloves garlic, minced
- 2 tablespoons fresh lemon juice
- 2 tablespoons extra virgin olive oil
- 1 tablespoon chopped fresh dill (or 1 teaspoon dried dill)
- Salt and pepper to taste

Instructions:

1. Start by grating the cucumber. Use a box grater or food processor to grate the cucumber. Once grated, place the cucumber in a fine-mesh sieve or colander set over a bowl. Sprinkle the grated cucumber with a little salt and let it sit for about 10-15 minutes to release excess moisture. Afterward, gently squeeze the grated cucumber to remove any remaining liquid.

2. In a mixing bowl, combine the grated cucumber, plain Greek yogurt, minced garlic, fresh lemon juice, extra virgin olive oil, and chopped fresh dill. Stir until all the ingredients are well combined.

3. Taste the tzatziki sauce and season with salt and pepper to taste. Adjust the seasoning as needed.

4. Cover the tzatziki sauce and refrigerate it for at least 1 hour before serving to allow the flavors to meld together.

5. Before serving, give the tzatziki sauce a quick stir. If desired, garnish with a drizzle of extra virgin olive oil and a sprinkle of fresh dill.

6. Serve the tzatziki sauce chilled as a delicious dip for pita bread, vegetables, or grilled meats, or use it as a flavorful condiment for gyros, sandwiches, or wraps.

Enjoy the fresh and tangy flavors of homemade tzatziki sauce! Adjust the consistency by adding more yogurt for a thicker sauce or a splash of water for a thinner sauce.

101. Turmeric

1. Turmeric Golden Milk Latte:
  - 1 cup milk (dairy or plant-based)
  - 1 teaspoon ground turmeric
  - 1/2 teaspoon ground cinnamon
  - 1/4 teaspoon ground ginger
  - Pinch of ground black pepper
  - Sweetener of choice (such as honey, maple syrup, or agave), to taste
  - Optional: 1/2 teaspoon vanilla extract

Instructions:
  1. In a small saucepan, heat the milk over medium heat until warm but not boiling.
  2. Whisk in the ground turmeric, ground cinnamon, ground ginger, ground black pepper, and sweetener of choice until well combined.
  3. Continue to heat the mixture, stirring occasionally, until warmed through and fragrant.
  4. Remove from heat and stir in the vanilla extract, if using.
  5. Pour the turmeric golden milk latte into mugs and enjoy immediately.

2. Turmeric Roasted Cauliflower:
  - 1 head cauliflower, cut into florets
  - 2 tablespoons olive oil
  - 1 teaspoon ground turmeric
  - 1/2 teaspoon ground cumin
  - 1/2 teaspoon ground coriander
  - Salt and pepper to taste
  - Fresh parsley or cilantro, chopped (for garnish)

Instructions:
  1. Preheat your oven to 400°F (200°C). Line a baking sheet with parchment paper or foil.
  2. In a large bowl, toss the cauliflower florets with olive oil, ground turmeric, ground cumin, ground coriander, salt, and pepper until evenly coated.
  3. Spread the seasoned cauliflower florets out in a single layer on the prepared baking sheet.
  4. Roast in the preheated oven for 25-30 minutes, or until the cauliflower is tender and golden brown, stirring halfway through cooking.
  5. Remove from the oven and transfer the roasted cauliflower to a serving dish.
  6. Garnish with chopped fresh parsley or cilantro before serving.

Enjoy these flavorful recipes featuring turmeric! Adjust the seasoning and spice level according to your preferences.

102. Ginger

1. Ginger Honey Lemon Tea:
  - 1-inch piece of fresh ginger, peeled and sliced
  - 1 tablespoon honey (or more to taste)
  - Juice of 1/2 lemon
  - 1 cup water

Instructions:
  1. In a small saucepan, bring the water to a boil.
  2. Add the sliced ginger to the boiling water and reduce the heat to low. Simmer for 5-10 minutes.
  3. Remove the saucepan from heat and let the ginger steep in the water for an additional 5 minutes.
  4. Strain the ginger-infused water into a mug.
  5. Stir in the honey and lemon juice until well combined.
  6. Enjoy your soothing ginger honey lemon tea hot.

2. Ginger Garlic Stir-Fry Sauce:
  - 1/4 cup soy sauce (or tamari for gluten-free)
  - 2 tablespoons rice vinegar
  - 1 tablespoon honey or maple syrup
  - 1 tablespoon minced fresh ginger
  - 2 cloves garlic, minced
  - 1 teaspoon sesame oil
  - 1 teaspoon cornstarch (optional, for thickening)

Instructions:
  1. In a small bowl, whisk together the soy sauce, rice vinegar, honey or maple syrup, minced ginger, minced garlic, and sesame oil.
  2. If you prefer a thicker sauce, you can mix in a teaspoon of cornstarch dissolved in a tablespoon of water.
  3. Use the ginger garlic stir-fry sauce to flavor your favorite stir-fry dishes with vegetables, tofu, chicken, shrimp, or beef. Simply add it to the stir-fry during the last few minutes of cooking and toss to coat.

Enjoy these delicious recipes featuring ginger! Adjust the ingredients and seasonings according to your taste preferences.

103. Cinnamon

1. Cinnamon Apple Oatmeal:
- 1 cup rolled oats
- 2 cups water or milk (dairy or plant-based)
- 1 apple, peeled, cored, and chopped
- 1 teaspoon ground cinnamon
- Pinch of salt
- Optional toppings: chopped nuts, dried fruit, maple syrup, or honey

Instructions:
1. In a saucepan, combine the rolled oats, water or milk, chopped apple, ground cinnamon, and a pinch of salt.
2. Bring the mixture to a boil over medium heat.
3. Reduce the heat to low and simmer, stirring occasionally, for 5-7 minutes, or until the oats are cooked and the mixture has thickened to your desired consistency.
4. Remove from heat and let the oatmeal sit for a minute or two to cool slightly.
5. Serve the cinnamon apple oatmeal hot, topped with your favorite toppings such as chopped nuts, dried fruit, maple syrup, or honey.

2. Cinnamon Roasted Sweet Potatoes:
- 2 large sweet potatoes, peeled and cubed
- 2 tablespoons olive oil
- 1 teaspoon ground cinnamon
- 1/2 teaspoon ground nutmeg
- Salt and pepper to taste

Instructions:
1. Preheat your oven to 400°F (200°C). Line a baking sheet with parchment paper or foil.
2. In a large bowl, toss the cubed sweet potatoes with olive oil, ground cinnamon, ground nutmeg, salt, and pepper until evenly coated.
3. Spread the seasoned sweet potatoes out in a single layer on the prepared baking sheet.
4. Roast in the preheated oven for 25-30 minutes, or until the sweet potatoes are tender and caramelized, stirring halfway through cooking.
5. Remove from the oven and transfer the roasted sweet potatoes to a serving dish.
6. Serve the cinnamon roasted sweet potatoes hot as a flavorful side dish.

Enjoy these delicious recipes featuring cinnamon! Adjust the ingredients and seasonings according to your taste preferences.

104. Cumin

1. Cumin-Spiced Black Bean Soup:
  - 2 tablespoons olive oil
  - 1 onion, chopped
  - 2 cloves garlic, minced
  - 2 teaspoons ground cumin
  - 1 teaspoon ground coriander
  - 1/2 teaspoon ground chili powder (optional)
  - 2 cans (15 ounces each) black beans, drained and rinsed
  - 4 cups vegetable or chicken broth
  - Salt and pepper to taste
  - Optional toppings: chopped fresh cilantro, diced avocado, sour cream, lime wedges

Instructions:

1. In a large pot, heat the olive oil over medium heat. Add the chopped onion and cook until softened, about 5 minutes.

2. Stir in the minced garlic, ground cumin, ground coriander, and ground chili powder (if using), and cook for another minute until fragrant.

3. Add the drained and rinsed black beans to the pot, along with the vegetable or chicken broth.

4. Bring the mixture to a boil, then reduce the heat to low and simmer for 15-20 minutes.

5. Use an immersion blender or transfer the soup to a blender and blend until smooth.

6. Season the soup with salt and pepper to taste.

7. Serve the cumin-spiced black bean soup hot, garnished with your favorite toppings such as chopped fresh cilantro, diced avocado, sour cream, and lime wedges.

3. Cumin-Spiced Roasted Vegetables:
  - Assorted vegetables (such as carrots, bell peppers, zucchini, cauliflower, and sweet potatoes), cut into bite-sized pieces
  - 2 tablespoons olive oil
  - 1 teaspoon ground cumin
  - 1/2 teaspoon ground coriander
  - 1/2 teaspoon smoked paprika
  - Salt and pepper to taste

Instructions:

1. Preheat your oven to 400°F (200°C). Line a baking sheet with parchment paper or foil.

2. In a large bowl, toss the bite-sized vegetables with olive oil, ground cumin, ground coriander, smoked paprika, salt, and pepper until evenly coated.

3. Spread the seasoned vegetables out in a single layer on the prepared baking sheet.

4. Roast in the preheated oven for 25-30 minutes, or until the vegetables are tender and caramelized, stirring halfway through cooking.

5. Remove from the oven and transfer the roasted vegetables to a serving dish.

6. Serve the cumin-spiced roasted vegetables hot as a flavorful side dish.

105. Oregano

Oregano and Lemon Roasted Chicken Thighs:
  - 4 bone-in, skin-on chicken thighs
  - 2 tablespoons olive oil
  - 2 cloves garlic, minced
  - 1 tablespoon dried oregano
  - Zest and juice of 1 lemon
  - Salt and pepper to taste

Instructions:
1. Preheat your oven to 400°F (200°C). Line a baking sheet with parchment paper or foil.

2. In a small bowl, whisk together the olive oil, minced garlic, dried oregano, lemon zest, lemon juice, salt, and pepper to make the marinade.

3. Place the chicken thighs on the prepared baking sheet. Rub the marinade all over the chicken thighs, ensuring they are evenly coated.

4. Roast in the preheated oven for 30-35 minutes, or until the chicken thighs are golden brown and cooked through, with an internal temperature of 165°F (75°C).

5. Remove from the oven and let the chicken thighs rest for a few minutes before serving.

6. Serve the oregano and lemon roasted chicken thighs hot, accompanied by your favorite side dishes.

Enjoy these delicious recipes featuring oregano! Adjust the ingredients and seasonings according to your taste preferences.

Dear Readers,

I want to extend my heartfelt gratitude to each and every one of you who embarked on the journey through "100+ Dishes of the Galveston Diet for Menopause." Your decision to explore this book is not just a testament to your commitment to your health but also a step towards embracing wellness in a holistic way.

Thank you for allowing my words to be a part of your quest for better health during this transformative phase of life. Your trust in the knowledge shared within these pages means the world to me. I hope that the recipes and insights offered have not only nourished your body but also empowered you to navigate menopause with grace and vitality.

As you continue along your wellness journey, remember that you are not alone. Whether you're experimenting with new recipes, adapting lifestyle changes, or simply seeking understanding, know that there is a community of support behind you.

Once again, thank you for choosing "100+ Dishes of the Galveston Diet for Menopause" and for being a part of this incredible journey. Here's to your health, happiness, and thriving through menopause and beyond!

With warm regards,